THE THEORY OF CHINESE MEDICINE

A Modern Interpretation

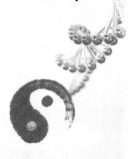

THE THEORY OF CHINESE MEDICINE

A Modern Interpretation

Hong Hai
Nanyang Technological University, Singapore

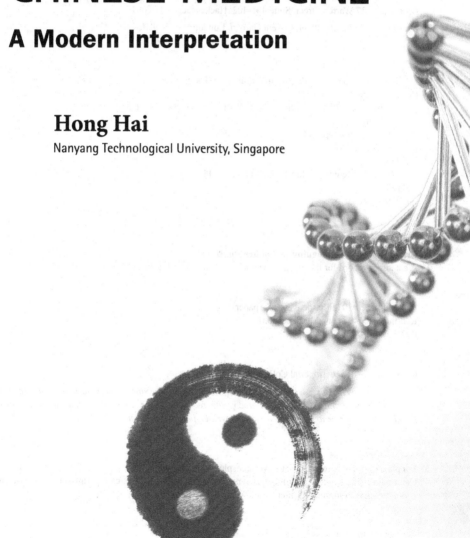

Imperial College Press

ICP

Published by

Imperial College Press
57 Shelton Street
Covent Garden
London WC2H 9HE

Distributed by

World Scientific Publishing Co. Pte. Ltd.
5 Toh Tuck Link, Singapore 596224
USA office: 27 Warren Street, Suite 401-402, Hackensack, NJ 07601
UK office: 57 Shelton Street, Covent Garden, London WC2H 9HE

Library of Congress Cataloging-in-Publication Data
Hong, Hai, 1943–   author.
    The theory of Chinese medicine : a modern interpretation / Hai Hong.
       p. ; cm.
    Includes bibliographical references and index.
    ISBN 978-1-78326-427-8 (hardcover : alk. paper)
    I. Title.
    [DNLM: 1. Medicine, Chinese Traditional. 2. Philosophy, Medical. 3. Qi. WB 55.C4]
    R127.1
    610.951--dc23
                                                                            2013042656

British Library Cataloguing-in-Publication Data
A catalogue record for this book is available from the British Library.

First published 2014 (hardcover : alk. paper)
Reprinted 2014 (in paperback edition)
ISBN 978-1-78326-448-3 (pbk)

Typeset by Stallion Press
Email: enquiries@stallionpress.com

Printed in Singapore

About the Author

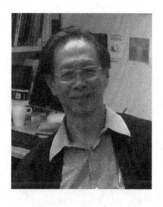

Hong Hai is Adjunct Professor and Senior Fellow at the Institute of Advanced Studies, Nanyang Technological University (NTU). Trained originally in engineering and economics, he had an earlier career as chief executive of a pharmaceutical company before studying Chinese medicine and the philosophy of science, graduating with an MD (Beijing University of Chinese Medicine), MPhil (Cambridge) and PhD (London). His doctoral dissertation examining the scientific basis for Chinese medical theory was written under the noted philosopher of science and medicine John Worrall.

Professor Hong Hai has chaired the Singapore parliamentary committee on health, and was a founding member of the Ministry of Health's TCM Practitioners Board and chairman of its academic committee. He practises medicine part-time at the Public Free Clinic and the Renhai Clinic, which he founded. As a pastime he started café Herbal Oasis which serves health teas and foods and hosts *salon-style* seminars on physical and social well-being.

Foreword

Donald Gillies

Traditional Chinese Medicine (TCM) has been criticised for being unscientific. This book discusses this criticism in detail. The author is not simply expounding TCM. He puts forward a particular interpretation of TCM, designed to overcome some of the difficulties, which have been detected in the system.

A fundamental problem is that some of the entities of TCM, such as the meridians, do not correspond to anything, which modern anatomists can observe, and internal organs have functions quite different from those assigned by modern physiology. The author tries to deal with this by developing what could be called an empiricist/pragmatist account of TCM. This reduces the entities postulated by TCM to observable functions, and TCM theory is interpreted as comprising heuristic models.

The author then goes to argue that TCM in his interpretation can be tested empirically using some of the methods of evidence-based medicine. The author develops his particular interpretation of TCM in a clear and rigorous fashion, and gives a thorough account of how TCM in this sense might be tested empirically. This is a book which should not be missed by anyone with an interest in Chinese medicine.

Donald Gillies is Emeritus Professor of Philosophy of Science and Mathematics in the Department of Science and Technology Studies at University College London. He has written extensively on the philosophy of science and the foundations of probability, and in recent years researched the application of philosophy of science to medicine.

Preface

Traditional Chinese Medicine (TCM) has been criticized by some scientists because the theory on which it is based involves abstract entities like *qi, jing* and 'meridians' that are ambiguous and ill-defined. The functions of the internal organs, which play such a crucial role in modern medical understanding of human physiology, are very different in TCM theory from those of modern physiology. For the example, the 'spleen' in TCM governs the entire digestion process, and the 'kidney' has functions in growth, sex and warming of the body. These notions are at odds with the functions of these organs in biomedicine.

Even harder to accept for the modern scientist are TCM methods of therapy that are based on the *yin-yang* principle, the model of the five elements, and the classification of illnesses according to standard constellations of symptoms (TCM '*syndromes*'). The validity of these methods and their usefulness for therapy has yet to be satisfactorily proven by the methods of modern evidence-based medicine.

This book takes the view that TCM may have an important contribution to make to health care, both as a form of complementary medicine supporting biomedical medicine and also as an alternative system of therapy for a range of illnesses. However, it suggests that for TCM to be understood and accepted by scientists in these roles, it is necessary to reconstruct TCM theory by:

(a) Providing explanations of TCM entities as abstractions and constructs that relate to observable body functions and illness symptoms and
(b) Interpreting TCM theory as comprising heuristic models that were constructed from clinical experience to fit empirical observations of illnesses and their treatments by TCM methods.

Such a reconstruction of TCM theory would not in the main violate the main tenets of Chinese medical theory, but should interpret its concepts and principles in a manner that avoids the alleged Kuhnian incommensurability of Chinese and Western systems of medicine.

Scientists should be less concerned with the ontological status of TCM entities and the epistemic credentials of TCM models than with the ability of these concepts and models to guide physicians in therapy. More importantly, the argument that these models are testable using the methods of evidence-based medicine can and should be made.

There are methodological difficulties associated with randomised controlled trials for TCM models, partly because TCM treatments tend to be individualised patient-centric and syndromes are dynamic in nature. Observational trials using past clinical data may be more appropriate in many situations. It is also possible that, for patients who are more culturally attuned to

TCM, the placebo effect is strongly at play and may render the real effects of TCM treatments harder to tease out in clinical trials. While these present real practical difficulties to the researcher, they are not insurmountable. Promising work is already in progress in both the East and West to test the efficacy of TCM methods.

A distinction is made between testing TCM theory and its methods of therapy on the one hand and clinical trials conducted on Chinese herbs for drug discovery purposes on the other. The former revolves around the differentiation of TCM syndromes and their treatment by TCM interventions such as herbal formulations and acupuncture. The latter applies modern biomedical pharmacology to botanical sources of drugs. Both are important, but the focus of the book is on the former.

Much useful work is being done on the latter by such bodies as the Consortium for the Globalisation of Chinese Medicine where important research is being conducted on to treat diseases. Its work lends credibility to the notion that some Chinese herbs have therapeutic value, but most of it should be regarded as pharmacological exploration of Chinese herbal sources of new drugs rather than a direct vindication of Chinese medical theory; in essence, these activities amount to little more than mining for new Western drugs from Chinese herbal sources.

The main postulates of TCM should be put to rigorous test. The result may be a leaner but more robust theory, with parts that do not stand up to the test being rejected or modified, and a possible acceptance of its more modest therapeutic claims for a limited range of pathological conditions such as pain and certain chronic illnesses and idiopathic conditions. A reconstructed TCM theory with more realistic claims backed by clinical trials may well provide a pragmatic and acceptable basis for the selective adoption of TCM interventions by modern physicians.

It is hoped that this book will make a contribution to a better understanding of Chinese medicine by the scientifically trained public and professionals in biomedicine who, befuddled by the ambiguities of TCM concepts and perplexed by the abstruse language of Chinese therapies, have either ignored or dismissed TCM and in so doing are the poorer for it.

Acknowledgments

The book is the outgrowth of research work over many years at the Beijing University of Chinese Medicine (BUCM), the Department of the History and Philosophy of Science (HPS) at Cambridge University, and the Department of Philosophy, Logic and Scientific Method at the London School of Economics (LSE).

My first exposures to Chinese medical literature in English were to Ted Kaptchuk's *The Web that has no Weaver* and Manfred Porkert's *Foundations of Chinese Medicine*. Both books greatly stimulated my interest in the subject but left me only partially satisfied, eventually leading me to research and offer the more scientifically pragmatic views in this book.

Kaptchuk's book is a brilliant introduction to the theory of Chinese medicine based on the traditional understanding of the subject, presented a little in the manner of religious apologetics, and has been an inspiration to generations of readers attempting to grasp the subtleties and intricacies of ancient medical thought. In my early studies of Chinese medicine, I was thrilled by his portrayal of Chinese theories as "a sensory image, a poetic exploration of what is going on."[1] Given my own background in the hard sciences, poetry provided a comforting refuge from the logic of

---

[1] Kaptchuk (2000:98).

the physical sciences, a reason to indulge in faith and imagery to explain how the abstractions of ancient medical thought somehow work usefully to treat illness. I believe Kaptchuk's approach is a good way for the general reader to start on a journey of understanding Chinese medicine. But faced with the imperatives of the scientific method espoused by the modern professional, I sought a more robust interpretation with which to respond to the criticism that biomedical scientists heap on the ambiguities of Chinese medical thought and the dearth of evidence for it.

I am indebted to the guidance of Professor John Worrall at LSE, whose views on clinical trials and certain issues in the philosophy of medicine have deeply influenced the content of this book, for which I nevertheless bear the sole responsibility. I also benefitted greatly from the seminars and classes at the philosophy department at LSE, where the influence of Karl Popper and Imre Lakatos was palpable.

I have gained from the profound insights into ancient Chinese medical thought of Professors Lu Zhaolin and Yan Jianhua at BUCM, and am thankful for the seminars and library resources at the Needham Research Institute and Sir Geoffrey Lloyd's lectures on ancient medicine at HPS, Cambridge. I am particularly grateful to my early teachers at the Singapore Institute of Chinese Medical Studies who kindled my midlife interest in Chinese medicine. I also gained from discussions of earlier drafts with various friends and colleagues, in particular the comments of Professors Donald Gillies at University College London and Peter Clark at the University of St Andrews.

My thanks go to Ms Joy Quek, senior editor at the Imperial College Press, who worked patiently on this manuscript and Professor KK Phua for his encouragement to publish this work.

Note on Terminology and Spelling

1. 'Herbs': Plant parts (roots, barks, seeds, etc.), minerals and animal parts used in Chinese medicine are collectively called '*materia medica*'. For convenience of reference, the term 'herbs' is used in this book to mean *materia medica*.

2. The *pinyin* system of spelling Chinese words, used as a standard in China, Singapore and increasingly in Western countries, is adopted instead of the older Wade–Giles system, used mainly in Taiwan today. '*Qi*' in *pinyin* is '*chi*' in the Wade–Giles system.

3. 'Regulate *qi*': This follows the common translation of *li qi* 理气, which means 'to assist in the flow of *qi*' in the body.

4. 'Syndrome': A TCM syndrome is a constellation of symptoms that define a pathological condition; also known as a 'pattern' or 'manifestation' (and it is similar to but conceptually different from the 'syndrome' in Western medicine).

5. 'Tonify' is not a term used in common English but standard in Chinese translation for 'provide a tonic for'; this meaning is adopted in this book.

Contents

Chapter 1

Chinese Medical Theory and its Rational Reconstruction

*The man who first saw the exterior of the box from above later
sees its interior from below.*

Thomas Kuhn

Traditional Chinese Medicine (TCM) has been charged with being unscientific because the theory on which it is based involves entities like *qi* (*chi*) and 'meridians' that appear ambiguous, and because the internal organs like the kidney and the spleen are understood very differently from those of modern anatomy and physiology. Furthermore, TCM methods of therapy based on the ancient principles of *yin-yang* and the five elements, as well as the classification of illnesses by constellations of symptoms known as TCM 'syndromes', are largely unproven by the clinical trial protocols of modern evidence-based medicine.

Do these conspicuous failings render the case for TCM as a credible system of medicine a hopeless one? Should TCM be relegated to the realm of murky human enterprises that attract a large followings because of a demonstrably strong placebo effect, appealing to the hopes and superstitions of believers whom mainstream has failed to heal?

This book makes the case that Chinese medicine is nothing more — and decidedly also nothing less — than a healing method based on somewhat crude and sometimes inaccurate empirical science developed over the centuries from clinical experience. Its theory comprises heuristic models, concepts and methods distilled from empirical observations that threw up an intricate system of diagnosis and a broad menu of herbal and acupuncture remedies. Through a review and interpretation of major parts of the theory, I shall explain how Chinese medicine can be considered scientific by examining the meanings and limitations of its theoretical claims. I outline the kind of clinical and pharmacological research that would be required to reconstruct TCM theory for better understanding by the scientific community.

In doing so, it is necessary to go beyond evidence from numerous clinical trials done in both the East and West demonstrating with varying degrees of success that certain acupuncture treatments do relieve pain and that some Chinese herbs have positive medicinal effects on specific diseases. For example, acupuncture is used extensively in the treatment of back, neck and shoulder pains[2]; the herb *mahuang* (*Herba Ephedrae*) is a source of ephedrine used in cold and allergy medications; the common herb *huangqi* (Astragalus) is a supplementary source of the body's telomerase used to promote cell regeneration.[3] Such observations do little more than indicate that Chinese medicine is a useful source for Western drug discovery and new interventions.

What needs to be demonstrated is not just anecdotes of TCM interventions yielding useful outcomes, but that TCM theory makes sense because it leads to systematic methods of diagnosis and therapeutic interventions that can alleviate and cure illnesses, as confirmed by clinical trials.

---

[2] Back and shoulder pains are among the conditions recognised as treatable by acupuncture by the World Health Organisation (2003).
[3] Kendrick (2009).

This book reconstructs TCM theory by: (a) providing explanations of TCM entities as abstractions and constructs that relate to observable body functions and illness symptoms and (b) interpreting TCM theory as comprising heuristic models that were constructed from clinical experience to fit empirical observations of illnesses and their treatments with herbal medications and acupuncture. It does not attempt to rewrite Chinese medical theory, but explains it by reinterpreting key concepts like *qi* and 'phlegm' and by elucidating the nature of TCM models. It suggests that scientists should be less concerned with the ontological status of TCM entities (i.e. whether they exist) and the epistemic credentials of TCM models (whether they are real or fictional) than with the ability of these concepts and models to guide physicians in therapy. More importantly, it makes the argument that these models are testable using the methods of evidence-based medicine.

I approach these tasks by focusing on some principal epistemological issues in the theory of Chinese medicine. Ultimately, the question is this: Is Chinese medicine based on science? In other words, is it genuinely testable and does it have an evidential basis so that it can be justifiably used for explanation and prediction?

A principal objective for this book is filling a gap in the academic and professional literature on Chinese medicine. While there is an extensive literature aimed at elucidating the mysteries of Chinese medicine and some piecemeal attempts at interpreting its concepts in biomedical terms,[4] little serious effort has been made to take an approach based on the philosophy of science to better understand Chinese medicine. Philosophy of science is the branch of philosophy that deals with the nature of science and scientific theories and examines the legitimacy of scientific methods for claiming discoveries of truth and knowledge. This book takes a

---

[4] See, for example, Porkett (1974) and Katpchuk (2000).

philosophy of science approach to evaluating TCM as a legitimate science and the nature of knowledge based on its theory.[5]

1.1 Chinese versus Western Medicine

In this book, Chinese medicine refers to the system of medicine that has been practised in China since ancient times. It is based on a body of theory that does not incorporate the scientific advances of Western medicine in modern times, in particular, the discoveries of microbiological agents like viruses and bacteria, as well as the enormous expansion in the understanding of human physiology and molecular biology since the advent of the Scientific Revolution in 17th century Europe. Chinese medicine, practised as an alternative to modern Western medicine in scientifically developed China and other East Asian countries, is as much an anachronism as would be ancient Greek and Galenic medicine were they to be practised in Europe today. Yet, in developed East Asian countries and some Western countries as well, it is indeed a serious alternative system taught in state-accredited university medical degree courses, complete with graduate and research programmes.

Chinese medicine was practised in China as mainstream medicine well into the second half of the 20th century. Following the large-scale introduction of Western science in the wake of the May 4th Movement of 1919 (the 'Chinese Enlightenment'),[6] Western medicine rapidly gained ground over Chinese medicine in public health care. By the 1970s, there were more Western physicians than Chinese physicians. Nonetheless, even today, Chinese

---

[5] The 20th century philosopher Ludwig Wittgenstein famously said that the aim of philosophy is to show the fly the way out of the fly bottle. In taking a philosophical perspective of Chinese medical theory, I am of the opinion that criticism by some scientists, that TCM entities are unobservable and unmeasurable, stems from treating them as physical entities rather than abstractions. That gets them into the fly bottle.
[6] Schwartz (1986).

medicine continues to play a significant role in health care, particularly in rural areas of the country.[7]

Controversy over the validity of Chinese medical theory and the case for continuing state support for it was an inevitable consequence of the May 4th Movement. Young nationalists, weary of a technologically backward China that suffered repeated incursions into its territories by Western powers following the Opium Wars in the mid-19th century, viewed the adoption of Western science and technology and democratic principles as the only way to revive the nation and restore its former glory.[8] Young scholars returning from universities in America, Europe and Japan saw Chinese medicine as a relic of China's scientifically backward past and mounted a campaign to eradicate it and replace it with Western medicine.

A public debate broke out in the 1920s when Yu Yan, who studied Western medicine in Japan, proposed the replacement of what he deemed unscientific Chinese medicine by Western medicine and the abolition of all Chinese medical practices other than the use of herbs, whose (alleged) therapeutic properties would be subject to research by clinical trials.[9] The robust response of the Chinese medical fraternity led initially by Yun Tieqiao set the stage for acrimonious debates that raged for over 20 years.[10] The conflict enjoyed a respite during the civil war followed by the ascendancy of Mao Zedong in the 1949 revolution. Mao, a believer in Chinese medicine but impressed also with the great advances made by Western science and medicine, declared

---

[7]In 1949, there were 38,000 Western and 276,000 Chinese physicians; by 1975, there were 292,980 and 228,640 respectively (WHO 1985:17).

[8]Schwartz (1986).

[9]Wang (2003) and Lei (2002).

[10]See Yu Yan (1933) and Yun Tieqiao (1922). The Chinese convention of stating the family name (surname) first is followed, thus, 'Yun' is Yun Tieqiao's surname.

Chinese medicine to be a "treasure trove of Chinese wisdom", ordered its modernisation and encouraged its integration with Western medicine. By edict, the training of doctors in Western medicine included courses in Chinese medicine. They were encouraged to use Chinese medicine in combination with Western methods, thereby lending a measure of scientific legitimacy to the former. Some observers interpret this as part of Mao's political agenda to show that the Chinese also had technology and knowledge from which the West could equally learn.[11]

The integration of Chinese and Western medicine began in earnest following Mao's lead. By the 1960s, colleges of Chinese medicine had been established and teams of scholars wrote textbooks in the modern Chinese language, systematically laying out the principles of Chinese medicine for the training of a new generation of Chinese doctors. These textbooks followed the style of Western medical books, each volume covering a specific area such as basic medical theory, pharmacology, diagnostic techniques, internal medicine, paediatrics, gynaecology, skin disorders and acupuncture. This method of studying medicine through standard texts was in contrast to the old way of learning from ancient medical classics, studying recorded cases of famous or legendary physicians and sitting as apprentices at the feet of experienced practitioners. As medical colleges grew and expanded, post-graduate degrees and extensive research programmes were introduced. Today dozens of Chinese medical universities and colleges turn out large numbers of doctoral dissertations and publications by Chinese as well as international research students from Japan, Korea, Singapore, Australia, Europe and the US.

The modernisation of Chinese medicine resulted in a systematisation of Chinese medical theory not to be found in the

---

[11] Taylor (2005:13–17,120).

classics, as well as additions to the theory that implicitly incorporated Western notions like viruses and bacteria (termed 'toxins') and borrowed concepts like the immune system and essential vitamins and minerals. The result of these sweeping changes was the birth of 'Traditional Chinese Medicine' (TCM), the modern form of Chinese medicine. TCM was traditional only in the sense that it kept intact the main core of ancient Chinese medical theory. In the rest of this book we use the term 'TCM theory' to refer to the modern systematised form of Chinese medical theory.

TCM attracted attention in the West following President Richard Nixon's historic visit to China in 1972. Western doctors saw Chinese medicine at work and witnessed the use of acupuncture to treat pain and as a form of anaesthesia. This aroused interest in TCM as a system of alternative or complementary medicine. In recent years, rising rates of serious illnesses like heart disease, strokes, cancer and diabetes, even as Western medicine made spectacular advances in knowledge and technology, may also have influenced patients to seek alternative methods of health care.

Sixty years after Mao's edict for Chinese and Western medicine to work together, the ideological differences between them have largely remained unresolved. Integration of TCM and Western medicine has taken place only to the limited extent that TCM physicians are sufficiently trained in Western medicine to use both systems of medicine in their clinical work, whilst Western-trained doctors take short courses to expose them to the basics of TCM. For the TCM physician, diagnosis by TCM methods is supplemented by laboratory tests and modern diagnostic procedures like blood tests, X-rays, MRIs and PET scans. The treatment administered could be a combination of Chinese herbs, acupuncture and selected Western pharmaceuticals such as antibiotics, steroids and anti-inflammatory drugs. These physicians think in TCM terms when they diagnose the *imbalances* underlying an illness and decide the therapies to be administered accordingly. They would be prepared to, and often do, supplement TCM treatments with Western drugs to address more urgent conditions, including antibiotics for bacterial infections and steroids for acute inflammations.

The term 'imbalance' is used here in the generic sense of abnormality or deviation from the healthy state of the body. The kind of imbalance in particular pathological conditions is more precisely defined by TCM as deficiencies in *yin* and *yang* and/or the presence of pathological conditions like heat, cold, dampness, phlegm and blood stasis. These terms are used in TCM in a different way from ordinary medical language and will be explained in subsequent chapters.

To illustrate the differences between the TCM and the modern Western medical approach to illness, take a common example of a patient who has just recovered from influenza. He is free of the virus but has a persistent cough with yellowish or greenish (bacterially infected) sputum, suffers from weakness and irritability, and feels dry in the throat and warm in the body even though his temperature is normal. His tongue is red, with a thick layer of yellowish cover (fur). From TCM diagnosis these are the classic symptoms of internal heat with warm phlegm.[12] Treatment consists of using 'cooling' herbs that, according to the Chinese pharmacopeia, reduce and eliminate internal heat, as well as other herbs that resolve phlegm. A week of herbal medication usually solves the problem but if the patient is run down and feeble it could take longer. At this stage, if the physician deems the patient to need assistance dealing with a bacterial infection, he may decide to prescribe a Western antibiotic to supplement

---

[12]'Heat' and 'phlegm', which have somewhat different usages in TCM theory from those in Western medicine, will be explained further in Chapter 4.

the herbal prescription.[13] After the cough and internal heat have subsided, a Chinese medical tonic may be prescribed to enhance the body's ability to restore balance and prevent a relapse.

The Western doctor would typically view the patient as having sputum in his respiratory system because of a secondary bacterial infection and the patient's feeling of body warmth and irritability merely as transient after-effects of the viral infection. The usual treatment would be a course of antibiotics to kill off the bacteria and an expectorant to deal with the sputum. It is not uncommon for such a condition to require repeat doses of antibiotics if the infection returns after the antibiotics are stopped. After the sputum dries up, a dry persistent cough often follows that could drag on for weeks.

TCM physicians in Asia often encounter such patients whose coughs have not recovered with Western medicine and therefore seek alternative treatments. There appears to be some anecdotal evidence that such patients find faster and more permanent relief with herbal treatments that aim at clearing heat and phlegm and rebalancing the body.

In this example, the TCM physician uses what he considers a holistic view of symptoms presented by the patient which enable him to draw conclusions about the nature of imbalance in the patient's body. In TCM parlance, the patient's imbalance is caused by internal heat and phlegm. This approach is different from that of Western medicine based on cellular biology, which aims at eliminating an offending microbiological pathogen (bacterium found in the sputum) and inducing the lungs to throw off the sputum that causes discomfort (this being the role of the expectorant).

---

[13] The combined use of Chinese and Western medicines is permitted in China but prohibited in most other jurisdictions, including Hong Kong, Singapore and Malaysia.

Can the two approaches be reconciled? It is tempting to give biomedical interpretations to the TCM medications. Perhaps the herbs have antibiotic and expectorant properties. Many Chinese herbs do indeed have antibiotic properties, but in forms too attenuated to be really effective in killing the bacteria involved. Herbs for resolving phlegm are deemed in TCM theory to have the effect of stopping the body from producing sputum rather than just expelling it. The modern TCM physician, drawing on his Western medical training, would view the bacterial infection as a consequence of the underlying imbalances in the body. The underlying condition (imbalances) is internal heat and phlegm. Its presence encourages secondary bacterial infection to take hold. Hence the real solution is not to kill the bacteria but remove the root of the problem, namely eliminate internal heat and phlegm and thereby restore balance. With internal balance restored, the body's own defences overcome the bacteria eventually. When the TCM physician adds the antibiotic, the aim is to assist weaker patients, particularly the elderly, whose body defences take too long or are inadequate for a satisfactory recovery. In this latter respect, the TCM physician's approach is not unlike that of more conservative Western physicians who would not prescribe antibiotics for a condition such as the one described above, except as a last resort for frail patients with life-threatening infections. The conservative doctor prefers the body to use its own immune system to overcome the infection, thereby strengthening it for future battles, but also reducing the incidence of bacteria mutating and becoming resistant to the antibiotic used.

Advocates of the TCM approach readily acknowledge the overwhelming superiority of Western science and modern medicine in unravelling the microbiological mechanisms by which disease affects physiological processes, as well as the drugs that destroy hostile pathogens and rectify cellular disorders. The TCM approach is to look at underlying conditions (imbalances) that allow the pathogens to take hold or the cellular disorders to arise. Thomas Kuhn's remark may not have been intended to be used in a medical context, but anyway seems to be pertinent here:

"The man who first saw the exterior of the box from above later sees its interior from below."[14]

TCM could be deemed as looking at the health of the human body holistically from above, whilst Western medicine looks at it from below, at the level of cells, genes and microbiological agents. This is of course not a fair characterisation of Western medical principles, which also encourage looking at the patient's body as a whole rather than just his or her blood tests and X-rays. But the reality is that Western medicine has been spoilt by great advances in diagnostic technology, so doctors tend to rely more on laboratory tests than on observation of symptoms presented by the patient on examination. The role of the family physician or general practitioner has also declined relative to that of the specialist. TCM has only direct visual and tactile observations, and the patient's description of how he feels, on which to rely, hence being holistic is its only choice.

Chinese diagnosis relies on directly observable symptoms presented by the patient, including the patient's own detailed description of how he feels, then proceeds to draw conclusions on how the body's condition has deviated from that of a healthy and balanced state. Therapy consists of bringing the body back to the balanced state. Like the ubiquitous wooden-wheeled cart pulled by a bullock in ancient China, Chinese medicine is technologically primitive. Like the bullock cart, it is crude and slow but sometimes gets the job done. Occasionally perhaps it even

---

[14] Kuhn (1970:111).

takes you through dirt tracks and hilly terrain that the BMW cannot handle.

Chinese medicine invented relatively simple models of the human body and of disease causation; it has applied these models in complicated ways to handle a wide variety of illnesses using experience that physicians gained over its long history. That many people were healed *when* these methods were applied should not be in doubt. What can legitimately be asked is whether they were healed *by* the methods applied. Would the same number have been healed anyway if nothing had been done? (Close to 100% of common colds heal with no medical treatment).

Even if the answer to this question is 'no', meaning that there are some patients who are healed by Chinese medicine who would not have been healed if nothing had been done, it can still legitimately be asked if the therapeutic gain was caused by something specific to the TCM treatment rather than by a placebo effect. Hence there is ultimately a need to put TCM therapeutic methods to the test through clinical trials.

1.2 Reconstructing TCM Theory

Attitudes towards TCM are virtually polarised into two camps: the believers and non-believers. Most TCM practitioners belong to the first camp. Most Western doctors belong to the second group although typically, whilst rejecting TCM theory, some observe that TCM interventions may produce therapeutic results, a point conceded even by one of alternative medicine's sternest critics.[15]

---

[15] Singh and Ernst (2008:328): "TCM is difficult to evaluate. Some elements may be effective for some conditions, while other elements (e.g. cupping) are unlikely to offer any benefit above placebo."

Many Western doctors now also believe in and practise acupuncture as a method of pain relief without necessarily accepting TCM theory's explanation for its efficacy. For example, the Singapore health ministry recognises a one-year part-time course to qualify Western doctors for the practice of acupuncture in their clinical work. These doctors learn to needle various acupoints for symptomatic relief of conditions such as pain, dizziness and insomnia; few of them believe the ancient Chinese theories that attempt to explain the therapeutic mechanism of acupuncture. (We shall return to this point in the discussion of 'Western acupuncture' in Chapter 7.)

TCM faces legitimate challenges by Western science on two counts. First, many of its core concepts like '*qi*', 'meridians' and 'phlegm' sound like meaningless or, at any rate, metaphysical entities, ill-defined and mostly not measurable and even unobservable. Second, the models used in TCM theory are mostly untested; it has also not been generally made clear that they are testable.

Borrowing a term from Lakatos' classic *The History of Science and its Rational Reconstruction*, a rational reconstruction of TCM theory would at the very least have to address the two core issues raised above. The proposed approach of this book is normative in the sense of the term used by Lakatos:

> [P}hilosophy of science provides normative methodologies in terms of which the historian reconstructs 'internal history' and thereby provides a rational explanation of the growth of objective knowledge.[16]

But it would also be helpful to the scientist trying to understand TCM theory to interpret it in the light of modern

---

[16]Lakatos (1970:91).

biomedical knowledge. This text suggests an approach based on the thesis that Chinese medical theory is derived from empirical observation and expressed through heuristic models.

TCM theory presents a number of problems for the scientist. It employs complex concepts like '*qi*' and 'phlegm' that have multiple and often somewhat obscure meanings. It reduces anatomy to: (a) a set of 'organs' that are in fact functional systems and not somatic structures as we understand them in modern anatomy and (b) a network of 'meridians' (channels) that have been painstakingly mapped out in medical manuals but have never been isolated in human dissections. Its account of human physiology reduces it to simplified models of relationships among organs, meridians and body fluids.

A system of medicine based on anatomical and physiological models so much at variance with modern medical knowledge of the human body cannot expect to be taken seriously unless there is evidence that — its apparently dubious theoretical base aside — it works as an effective tool of diagnosis and therapy for at least for some illnesses. Based on the history of Chinese medicine in providing health care from ancient to modern times, there is a *prima facie* case for supposing that it provides healing for *some* ailments. Any experienced doctor would concede that some folk remedies do work and that a few old wives' tales are true. There can be little doubt, for example, that the herb *dahuang* (*Radix et Rhizome Rhei*) used for constipation can induce purging, as anyone who takes a large dose would rapidly discover, or that *mahuang* (*Herba Ephedrae*) helps induce perspiration and alleviate fevers (its derivative ephedrine is now extensively used in Western cold medications).

But for most Chinese medical treatments, even when these treatments are followed by patient recovery, the question still remains whether the patient would have got better without treatment, or whether only a placebo effect was at work. Hence there is a need to study these treatments through appropriate clinical trials.

There is also the possibility that a treatment works for some but not for most of the ailments for which it makes claims. Bloodletting was practised in Chinese medicine and also in Europe, based on the now-defunct Galenic theory of body humours, for almost 2,000 years, before it fell into disrepute in the late 19th century. Yet it is used by modern medicine today as a life-saving method of treatment for a very limited number of blood-related illnesses such as hemochromatosis and *polycythemia rubra vera*.[17] Bloodletting (therapeutic phlebotomy) is used to treat hereditary hemochromatosis in which there is slow excessive iron build-up in the body, causing damage to organs such as the liver, heart and joints. Regularly reducing the volume of blood in the body is also currently the main treatment for *polycythemia rubra vera* in which the blood becomes much too thick, increasing the risk of clots and strokes. Phlebotomy can also help people who are producing too many red cells because their bodies are starved of oxygen owing to a heart or lung problem.

A small amount of bloodletting can (and is still used by some Chinese physicians) to temporarily relieve conditions like hypertension although, with the availability of modern drugs, this has now come to be regarded as a primitive and risky (infection-prone) method of treatment. The challenge then, for believers in TCM, is to tease out those conditions for which they can be demonstrated through clinical trials to work consistently.

TCM is not unlike Hippocratic and Galenic medicine practised in ancient Greece and Rome and medieval Europe, except that the Chinese continued using it to modern times and arguably may well have developed a better system. It is worthy of note that in modern Europe, enough useful knowledge in Galen's works

---

[17] Barton (2009) and Mestel (2001).

were considered to exist so these works continued to be studied in medical schools in England in the first half of the 20th century, in part because some of Galen's methods were still valid and useful. Likewise, TCM theory's main concepts and simple models may have captured some essential aspects of human physiology in some fuzzy holistic way such that it works for some ailments.

How consistently TCM works and for what medical conditions it works well could largely be a matter of perception. Chinese physicians reinforce their faith in these methods with anecdotal evidence of patients getting better with these treatments, unaware of or choosing to ignore the possibility of the *post hoc ergo propter hoc* fallacy.[18] But for the scientific community at large, appropriate clinical trials are needed to establish belief in these methods. What constitutes appropriate clinical trials will be one of the principal topics of this book.

The rational reconstruction of TCM theory would require not only the scientific interpretation of TCM concepts but also that it renders the explanations and predictions of TCM models testable by the methods of evidence-based medicine. It should show how it would be possible to conduct appropriate clinical trials to test the diagnosis and therapies prescribed by the theory. Such clinical trials should be expected to eventually reject some parts of TCM theory, modify others, and increase faith in those that are validated.

Such a reconstruction would represent a departure from received TCM theory taught in college texts for Chinese medical students. Received TCM theory is presented in these texts as immutable truths, somewhat like the laws of physics and chemistry, accurately reflecting underlying realities into which the

---

[18] The *post hoc ergo propter hoc* fallacy is the assumption that the patient gets better as a result of the treatment when in fact he recovers as a natural progression of the disease (which normally happens with an ailment like the common cold).

ancients had special insights, enabling them to put together an internally consistent set of concepts and models from which are derived the principles governing health and illnesses. Confronted with charges of lacking scientific proof for these principles, and appearing divorced from the reality with vague concepts like *qi*, phlegm and vital organs with functions radically different from those as by modern and physiology, a common defence has been that this is a system derived from the undoubted wisdom of ancient Chinese philosophy.[19] Naturally this cuts no ice with modern scientists, including those who might appreciate some aspects of Chinese philosophy but see no proven link between ancient philosophy and modern physiology.

When Kuhn's *Structure of Scientific Revolutions* appeared, besieged TCM theorists found a life raft in the idea of *incommensurability*. In Kuhn's pathbreaking account of paradigms in the history of scientific revolutions, a paradigm shift occurs when one theory replaces another, for example when Copernicus' heliocentric model of the solar system supplanted Ptolemy's model of an immovable earth at the centre of the universe, around which revolved the moon, sun and all other planets; or when Einstein's general theory of relativity replaced Newtonian theory. The pre-revolutionary and post-revolutionary paradigms are said to be incommensurable in the sense that the terms of one theory cannot be strictly translated into the terms of the other theory. Kuhn further clarified the notion of untranslatability using the idea that the lexical structures of two incommensurable theories cannot be mapped into each other.[20]

---

[19] For example, Liu (2003).

[20] Kuhn (1970). Psillos (2007), 115 comments, "Kuhn supplemented this notion of untranslatability with the notion of lexical structure: two theories are incommensurable if their lexical structures (i.e. their taxonomies of natural kinds) cannot be mapped into each other."

   Some advocates of Chinese medicines seized upon the idea of incommensurability to justify their position that TCM theories cannot be evaluated by evidence-based medicine criteria set by Western medicine. What resulted was that the dialogue between the two sides was effectively cut off, sometimes with exasperated antagonists resorting to name-calling when their arguments failed to convince their rivals.[21]

   The rest of this book explains why this longstanding dispute between Chinese and Western medicine thinkers is quite unnecessary. Resolution of the dispute needs them to understand the epistemological nature of TCM concepts and theories, and come to realise that some of these theories can indeed to put the test through appropriate clinical trials.

---

[21] For example, TCM concepts were called "gobbledygook" in "Dangerous Science taught at Middlesex University", see DCScience (2010); charges of "quackery" were made by Western doctors objecting to alternative medicine being taught at Australian universities, eliciting retorts of Western medical "dogmatism" (*The Straits Times*, 4th February 2012). Even less elegant language is common when Western medical scientists debate Chinese medical theorists at conferences.

Chapter 2

Chinese and Western Medical Thought: History and Issues

When many different diseases appear at the same time, it is plain that the
regimen is responsible in individual cases.

Hippocratic Writings

The core theory and concepts in TCM were developed when very little was understood about human anatomy and physiology. Unlike Greece and Rome in antiquity, ancient China forbade dissections as the human body was considered sacred. Ancient Chinese descriptions of the organs in the human body and substances contained therein were therefore simplistic and often conjectural. However the theory built around these entities became more complex in order to explain observable physiological phenomena, diagnose illnesses, prescribe therapies and contend with complications of changing symptoms as illnesses progress.

Essentially, TCM theory consists of a number of idealised models within which entities and concepts, and their mutual relationships, are presented in a manner that renders them applicable to the diagnosis and treatment of illnesses.

The TCM picture of the human body is highly simplified: besides skin, bone and connective tissue, the body comprises organs, three basic fluids (*qi*, blood and *jingye*), and pathways (meridians or channels) along which *qi* and other entities can travel.

19

The healthy body is one in which there is internal balance and normal flow of fluids and energy. Illness is expressed as a condition, or conditions, under which these flows are impeded and/or a number of entities are not in balance. Such pathological conditions are known in TCM as *syndromes*. Syndromes in TCM have some similarity to syndromes in Western medicine in that they comprise a number of typical or defining symptoms forming a distinct clinical picture indicative of a particular underlying disorder. The underlying disorder is presumed in Western medicine to be attributable to micro-organisms like virus, bacteria and fungi, unusual cellular behaviour, a dysfunctional immune system, abnormal endocrinal secretions, and the like, or a combination of these. For example, the irritable bowel syndrome (IBS) is exhibited as recurrent dyspepsia, abdominal pain and irregular bowel movements, the cause of which is unknown. The treatment is largely one of providing symptomatic relief. In TCM the syndrome of 'weak spleen and stomach *qi*' exhibits similar symptoms to that of IBS. The treatment addresses the underlying imbalance by providing a tonic for *qi* and promoting its flow.

The basic causes of illness are classified into external pathogenic and internal pathogenic factors. External factors comprise mainly climatic influences (heat, cold, dampness, dryness, wind, summer 'fire') that can invade the body. Internal factors comprise harmful emotions and improper living habits. External and internal pathogenic factors upset balance and interrupt smooth flows in the body, causing illness.

TCM models can thus be seen as attempts to explain the pathological conditions underlying illnesses. Diagnosis and therapy then consists of identifying these pathological conditions and finding matching therapies for them. This approach is known *differentiating the syndrome* and applying appropriate therapy, known as *bianzhenglunzhi* 辨证论治.

The core approach of TCM treatment of illness is thus basically directed at re-establishing balance and unimpeded flows, rather than at eliminating germs or correcting abnormal cell behaviour of cells as is the case for modern biomedicine. In a nutshell, TCM treatment is directed at resolving syndromes rather than overcoming disease, the *raison d'être* being that eliminating the syndrome takes away the basis for the continuation of the disease.[22]

2.1 Evolution of TCM Theory

Chinese and Greek medicines in distant antiquity were both dominated by the belief that illnesses were caused by spirits and demons, thus cures required the intervention of mediums or deities. In the practice of 'temple medicine' in ancient Greece, patients slept in temples so that the gods could appear in their dreams to heal their illnesses.

In China, a paradigm shift occurred with the appearance of what came to be regarded as the greatest of all Chinese medical classics, *The Huangdi Neijing* 黄帝内经 ('*Neijing*'), also known as

---

[22] A useful comparison with Western medicine can perhaps be drawn from treatment of malignant tumours. Chemotherapy kills cancer cells using chemical substances which are also toxic to normal cells albeit to different degrees. Radiation therapy destroys cancer cells in a targeted way by focusing radiation on the tumour and surrounding areas. Its effect on normal cells can be devastating: radiation therapy for brain tumours for example can usually be done only once, as brain cells undergo irreversible changes from the effect of radiation and usually may not withstand further rounds of radiation. TCM has no effective direct way of attacking the tumour. The closest that TCM medications come to addressing a malignant tumour is that some TCM herbs have anti-angiogenesis effects, reducing or cutting off the blood supply to tumours, causing them to shrink. Many Chinese herbs have been found to have anti-angiogenesis properties and there is much current pharmacological work discovering anti-angiogenesis drugs from herbal sources. See, for example, Wang *et al.* (2004).

The Yellow Emperor's Canon of Medicine, written in the Han dynasty (206 BC–220 AD).[23] The *Neijing* was the distillation of ideas and knowledge compiled over several hundred years by many scholars. Although its origin is attributed to the Han dynasty, it was continually refined, edited and expanded right up to China's final imperial dynasty, the Qing (1644 – 1911). Hence many editions of the *Neijing* exist. The Wang edition commonly used as a reference manual was compiled in the Tang dynasty (618–907).

The *Neijing* made a break with previous medical thought by refusing to attribute disease causation to numinous agents. It focused instead on environmental conditions and emotional factors and emphasised the importance of natural laws in the explanation of illnesses.[24] In particular, the *Neijing* brought to Chinese medicine the ideology of "systematic correspondence" by which all tangible and abstract phenomena could be categorised as manifestations of theoretical models of the human body (notably the *yin-yang* principle and the 'five-element model').[25] The descriptions of anatomical and physiological systems in the body, which include five pairs of vital organs (*zangxiang* 臟象), acupuncture meridians (*jingluo* 经络) (also known as channels and collaterals), and the key entities of '*qi*', 'blood' and 'body fluids', were understood in relation to these models.

Different schools of thought introduced interpretations and extensions of medical theory in the *Neijing*. These schools flourished

---

[23]"The Yellow Emperor" is an inept translation of *Huangdi*, the name of *Huang* emperor ('*di*'). 'Huang' has two usages — it is the colour yellow and it is a common surname in China. There was nothing yellow about the legendary emperor *Huangdi*, not any more than former British Prime Minister Gordon Brown had to do with the colour brown. He would (not) be amused at being called 'The Brown PM'.

[24]Unschuld (2003: 319).

[25]Unschuld (1985:5, 54).

from the Han dynasty to modern times, although in essence they did not depart from the core models of the *Neijing*.[26] Among the earliest of these schools was that based on *The Treatise on Febrile Diseases* (*Shanghan Lun* 伤寒论) by Zhang Zhongjing (150–219), which postulated that the harm caused by climatic influences such as cold, wind and dampness travelled along meridians and brought about progressive changes of body state (pathogenesis).

During the Song dynasty (960–1279), ideas from neo-Confucianism, Taoism and Buddhism stimulated the development of new medical doctrines. There followed vigorous contention among 'a hundred schools' of medical thought. Among the influential schools were those associated with Liu Yuansu (1120–1200) who founded the 'school of cooling' (*hanliang pai* 寒凉派), stressing the elimination of excess 'internal heat'; Li Gao (1180–1251) who regarded the digestive system as the fundamental basis for good health, hence founding the 'spleen–stomach school' (*piwei pai* 脾胃派); and Zhu Danxi (1281–1358) who founded the '*yin*-nourishing school' (*ziyin pai* 滋阴派) which claimed that man's body by nature tends to be deficient in *yin*, hence nourishing *yin* must be the basis of good health.

These contending schools introduced differing emphases in Chinese medicine that were in tune with the times and places in which they flourished. For example, the *yin*-nourishing school of Zhu Danxi was influential in the Yuan dynasty among wealthy officials who over-indulged in food and sex, which was thought to harm the *yin* of their kidneys, hence the need to nourish *yin*.

Late Ming and early Qing saw further development of medical thought, notably studies of infectious diseases common in

---

[26] Ren Yinqiu (1986:5–6), who started the study of "schools of thought in medicine" (中医各家学说) in the 1950s, emphasises that contending schools did not depart from the core models of the *Neijing*.

spring and summer in the south by the 'warm disorders school' (*wenbing xuepai* 温病学派) led by Wu Youxing (1582–1652). This was in contrast to the 'cold-damage model' of the *Shanghan Lun,* written by northerners of the Han dynasty who endured harsh winters and developed more robust constitutions, in contrast to those of "delicate southerners".[27] The *Shanghan* school consequently focused on disorders originating from exposure to cold and wind and their pathogenesis, whilst the *Wenbing* school were more concerned with infectious diseases and epidemics that broke out in the summer months in the south.

The first serious challenge to ancient Chinese medical theory was influenced by philosophical trends similar to those associated with the logical positivists and Karl Popper in Vienna. Like the logical positivists, Western-trained scholars like Yu Yan deemed unobservables in Chinese medicine as metaphysical and hence meaningless.[28] They regarded Chinese medical theory to be unfalsifiable and therefore unscientific. In defence, Chinese physicians cited extensive historical clinical records of successful treatments using Chinese medicine. In addition they appealed to the authority of ancient Chinese philosophy on which medical theory was based. The clinical record of Chinese medicine was difficult for Western doctors to dismiss, as many of them acknowledged the widespread existence of *prima facie* evidence of the efficacy of some Chinese medications and of acupuncture. But they insisted that the efficacy of Chinese methods be subjected to formal testing in accordance with the rigours of Western scientific tradition. As to invoking the wisdom of an ancient philosophical system to justify medical theory, this convinced few detractors as it was seen as merely shifting the burden of proof

---

[27] Hanson (2001: 262–292).
[28] Yu (1933).

from medicine to ancient philosophy and implicitly admitting its scientific inadequacy.

Following Mao's decision to modernise Chinese medicine, the first national textbook for instruction in TCM appeared in 1958, entitled *Outline of Chinese Medicine* (*Zhongyixue Gailun* 中医学概论).[29] Subsequent texts, covering different subjects within medicine, displayed deliberate similarity to their Western counterparts and they constituted a massive and unprecedented systematisation of Chinese medical theory and practice. Regulation of TCM practice was introduced through the licensing of medical practitioners at the state level with common national examinations. Since modernisation, TCM universities in China have required about 30–40% of the student's time to be spent on studying Western medicine. Graduates can practise basic Western medicine in addition to TCM. They can read modern diagnostic test results, prescribe Western drugs and perform simple surgical procedures. Research publications in TCM have yet to catch up in terms of rigour and methodology with those in the West, but their increasing numbers and improving quality attest to the recognition by TCM scholars that their theories and therapeutic methods should be put to tests similar to those used in evidence-based medicine.

Referring to the systematisation of Chinese medicine, Sivin opines that such change had been "most decisive over the past generation, with unmistakable influence from modern medicine".[30] Scheid notes that the transition was not without its controversies and contends that despite the apparent uniformity forced upon the TCM community by state-sanctioned textbooks and clinical

---

[29] Scheid (2002:74). A 1972 text *The Revised Outline of Chinese Medicine* 新编中医学概要 was translated into English by Sivin (1987).
[30] Sivin (1987:124).

practices, there remained a plurality of views among scholars and practitioners. Scheid's observation is especially pertinent considering that conservative scholars like Liu Lihong continue to regard the classics as the ultimate authority on medicine despite their formal training in TCM as the modern systematised form of Chinese medicine. They treat TCM as the product of adulteration and distortion by Western interpretation. Such conservatives seem to be a dying breed.[31]

As much as the systematisation of Chinese medicine was considered a radical transformation in the 1960s, the truth of the matter is that Chinese medical thought has largely stagnated since the emergence of the *Neijing*, as if time has virtually stood still after the theoretical breakthroughs of the Han dynasty. Indeed, generations of modern scholars of Chinese medicine have continued to treat the *Neijing* as the source of all Chinese medical wisdom. Among conservative scholars, the presumption is that the ancients were gifted with special powers of discernment which allowed them to see ultimate truths in medicine and record them accurately in the classics. Understanding these ultimate truths would be all it takes to grasp the theory of Chinese medicine although an enormous amount of scholarly work has to be invested in interpreting these ancient writings, not unlike research on ancient scriptures.

2.2 Diseases in Western Medical Thought

The history of Western medicine in ancient times was similar to that of Chinese medicine, but took a very different route in modern times. Knowledge would come from challenging accepted truths of the past and progress from scientific revolutions that

---

[31] Liu (2003).

challenged and replaced old theories and the pathbreaking discoveries following the advent of scientific medicine in 19th century Europe.[32]

Western medicine in distant antiquity evolved from spiritual beliefs but underwent a transformation similar to that brought to Chinese medicine by the *Neijing*. After the *Hippocrates Corpus* (circa 350 BC), diseases previously thought to be linked to spirits and gods were regarded as disorders caused either by external environmental factors or internal disruptions in the body. *The Nature of Man* (in *Hippocratic Writings*), for example, states:

> When a large number of people all catch the same disease at the same time, the cause must be ascribed to something common to all and which they all use; in other words to what they all breathe...However, when many different diseases appear at the same time, it is plain that the regimen [that is, diet and exercise] is responsible in individual cases.[33]

This insight led to the distinction in modern medicine between diseases caused by infectious and environmental factors and illnesses caused by factors internal to the body.

An influential medical sect, the Methodists, introduced a new medical theory that dominated the Roman world for some three centuries from Themison (123–143 BC) to the time of the emperor Marcus Aurelius (161–180 AD).[34] Hippocratic medicine had earlier tied together the part affected by disease and the etiological theory to explain the disease, thereby allowing the physician to ascertain indications for therapy based on the locus

---

[32] Porter (1997:XI).
[33] Lloyd (1983: 22–23).
[34] Nutton (2004:188).

of the disease.[35] The Methodists rejected this epistemological approach and insisted that good medicine was simply effective therapeutic practice and it was not necessary to search for the hidden causes of disease.[36] Thus Methodists spoke of 'affections' (*pathe*) rather than disease (*nosoi*) and did not concern themselves with etiology, convinced as they were that a good doctor should never concern himself with the causes of disease.[37] The Methodists emphasised notions of *repletion*, indicating excesses in the body, and *depletion*, indicating deficiencies. These notions were somewhat similar to excess (*shi*) and deficiency (*xu*) *syndromes* in Chinese medicine (see Chapter 6).

Galen (129–216 CE), whose ideas were to dominate Europe up to the end of the 16th century, rejected much of Methodism but his view of human health was in principle not all that different. Drawing inspiration from Aristotle and the *Hippocratic Writings*, he viewed organised human bodies, like bodies in nature, as composed of the four elements of fire, water, earth and air, with the four qualities of these four elements being heat, moisture, dryness and cold. Disease stemmed from abundance, scarcity or change taking place in the humours, comprising blood, phlegm, and yellow and black bile. Hence diseases were classified according to the humour that was in excess, or scarce, or which suffered a defect in its movements, each of which requiring a different therapeutic approach.[38] Such notions of excess and deficiency were to persist in Western medical thought right through to modern times, when their importance was eclipsed by notions of disease causation derived from discoveries

---

[35] Tecusan (2004:10).
[36] Nutton (2004:190).
[37] Tecusan (2004:4,10–11).
[38] Nutton (2004:202–215); Cumston (1926:137).

in microbiology. That such notions continue to be central to Chinese medical thought is worthy of note. It is as if the dazzling discoveries of microbiology diverted Western medical science to cells and genes and held it on the nosological track, neglecting the perspective of the body as a whole in relation to its internal and external environments. Chinese medicine on the other hand knew no microbiology and had little choice but to look at the body's external manifestations as a whole.

Ancient and pre-modern medicine in Europe focused on understanding the conditions of human bodies in the grip of disease, the progression of these conditions (pathogenesis), and appropriate therapies for healing. Less emphasis was placed on epistemological issues of causation — what made the patient fall ill in the first place. Before the 19th century, etiological discussions of disease in Europe revolved largely around moral and social factors such as drunkenness, intemperance, gluttony, and dissipation. Bardsley (1845), for example, attributed diabetes to indulgence in excessive amounts of cold fluid, poor living, sleeping at night in the open air in a state of intoxication, sudden halting of perspiration, and mental anxiety.

The Scientific Revolution of 16–17th century Europe laid the groundwork for the systematic merging of the classical and experimental sciences in the 19th century such as the transformation of the Baconian science of heat into an experimental-mathematical thermodynamics.[39] By the second half of the 19th century, systematic experimentation took root in medicine, particularly in physiology, and the profession of medicine gained new institutional forms and enhanced intellectual standards as it leveraged state resources for scientific research.[40] Hospitals moved from Church

---

[39] See Kuhn (1977:63).
[40] Kuhn (1977:60).

to State, and the emergence of hospital medicine (first in Paris) was characterised by scientific observation, pathological examination and a detailed knowledge of anatomy. The shift from a stress on Galenic holistic views of humeral balance to the new "anatomico-pathological" model would eventually lead to the discoveries of modern etiology.[41]

A major step forward was made with research on childbed fever (*puerperal sepsis*) in 1846 when Semmelweis observed that the mortality rates of women after childbirth varied with hygiene conditions, leading him to the conclusion that childbed fever was caused by decaying matter. Semmelweis used a hypothesis-testing methodology to infer that childbed fever was caused by "cadaveric matter" transmitted by doctors and students conducting autopsies in the hospital.[42]

Some 40 years later, a monocausal model of disease was proposed by Pasteur and Koch who had earlier isolated the *tubercle bacillus*. The *Henle-Koch Postulates* stated that a parasite "occurred in every case of the disease in question and occurred in no other disease as a fortuitous and non-pathogenic parasite", in effect insisting on a one-to-one correspondence between disease and parasite.[43] Koch called this approach to disease causation "the etiological standpoint".[44]

By the beginning of the 20th century, the etiological standpoint drove much of medical research. Bacteriology opened up the vision of finding biological agents to destroy them and eventually to the development of the antibiotic penicillin through the work of Fleming and Florey.[45] The use of antibiotics to combat

---

[41] Porter (1999:306).
[42] Hempel (1966:3–8); von Gyory (1905:94).
[43] Evans (1993:30).
[44] Carter (2003:1).
[45] Porter (1997:454–457).

disease-causing bacteria was a radical departure from Galenic (and Chinese) medicine that used medications only to restore balance and resolve internal obstructions.

However, other important diseases defied such straightforward etiological explanations. One such disease was beriberi, whose cause required a new deficiency theory of disease. The etiological standpoint had to be widened to include deficiency of certain organic chemicals essential to the body. Viruses presented a new set of problems. When viruses were involved, medical scientists found that causes of disease were more complex than could be explained by the simple etiological standpoint. For example, rhinoviruses are associated with only 20–25% of the common cold syndrome and are active mostly in the autumn. Furthermore, many viral infections are asymptomatic. Viruses are also thought to be linked to some forms of cancer, but seem to be neither necessary nor sufficient for the cancers to occur. Looking at the broad range of diseases, a single cause can result in a spectrum of clinical syndromes, and the same effect could result from several different causes, depending on the nature of the causative agent, the environment in which it operates, and the characteristics of the involved host. In the case of chronic (non-infectious) illnesses like heart disease, the complexity is such that epidemiologists prefer to talk about risk factors rather than causes.[46]

The situation is even murkier with subclinical epidemiology. Subclinical illnesses in which the patient experiences no obvious symptoms occur not only in infectious diseases, when infection occurs without disease, but also in chronic diseases. Many of the causes of disease are so ubiquitous that almost everyone has been exposed to them, and it is often not clear what makes disease

---

[46] Evans (1993:1, 46, 107).

develop in some but not in others. As the noted epidemiologist Alfred Evans puts it, it is the search for a "clinical illness promotion factor" for a given disease that poses the real challenge. He calls this the "third ingredient" in disease causation, in addition to microbiological agents and deficiencies in the body. [47]

The difficulties in the meaning of disease causation arise in part from the notion of causation itself, hence it is helpful to refer to philosophical discussions of causation and consider its relevance to disease causation and to the TCM view of illness and health.

2.3 Causation in Western Medicine

The etiological standpoint attributable to Henle and Koch was based on what Henle termed "necessary and universal causes", by which he meant that a cause must always have the same effect; the cause must also be necessary for its effect.[48] Applied to the *tubercle bacillus* discovered by Koch, this implied that anyone suffering from tuberculosis would have the *tubercle bacillus* in his body, and anyone with that bacillus in his system would suffer from tuberculosis; that is, the *tubercle bacillus* was necessary and sufficient for contracting tuberculosis. Henle seemed to want to use this to characterise disease causation in general, but there was an unsatisfactory narrowness in his notion of causality. This was evident when he criticised doctors in the following passage:

> Only in medicine are there causes that have hundreds of consequences or that can, on arbitrary occasions, remain entirely without effect. Only in medicine can the same effect flow from the most

---

[47] Evans (1993:213).
[48] Henle (1844).

varied possible sources...For almost every disease, after a specific cause or the admission that such a cause is not yet known, one finds the same horde of harmful influences — poor housing and clothing, liquor and sex, hunger and anxiety. This is just as scientific as if a physicist were to teach that bodies fall because boards or beams are removed...[49]

Henle approved of the approach of physicists who sought a single common cause (gravitation) to explain each instance of a class of similar events (falling bodies) and felt that rational medicine should do the same. He criticised medical researchers of his time for attributing causation to events that immediately preceded the event instead of following physicists in seeking universal scientific principles like gravitation.

One could argue that the Henle–Koch etiological standpoint often commits a similar sin. For example, the bacillus that 'causes' tuberculosis has an immediately preceding status, similar to that of the removal of a board preceding the fall of a body.

I would argue that it is more pertinent in Henle's example of falling bodies to identify the *motivation* for identifying the cause of the fall. Depending on the motivation, the questions of who removed the board, and for what purpose, would be natural ones to ask. Indeed, if the falling body was that of a human being working on a construction site and the courts were trying the case of homicide after someone removed the board on which the victim stood, no prosecutor in court would charge Newtonian gravitation with the crime. If an act of sabotage was involved in the removal of the board, the cause of the fall, for purposes of ascribing reprehensibility and meting out punishment, would be the wilful removal of the board by the saboteur.

---

[49] Cited in Carter (2003:25).

Henle's inept choice of example for disease causation is symptomatic of the fact that the literatures of medicine and philosophy of science rarely intersect, even though accounts of causation in the philosophy of science potentially could help elucidate the nature of disease causation. Consequently the notion of disease causation is a subject with which modern epidemiologists have expressed difficulty. Stehbens, for example, laments that:

> [At] the crux of the issue is the use and meaning of *cause* in medicine . . . If epidemiology continues to disregard the misusage (sic) of terminology . . . it threatens the very survival of logic and science in medicine.[50]

Carter declares that it is "totally pointless, hopeless and downright silly to think one can ever state precisely what it is for one thing to cause another".[51] As a matter of fact, the philosophical problem posed by Koch, Henle, Carter and others arises from focusing on necessary causes and not paying enough attention to sufficient causes.

I argue below that a necessary cause is often better viewed as the *definition* of the disease rather than its cause. For example, the presence of the *tubercle bacillus* in the body merely defines tuberculosis as a disease: a person in whom the *tubercle bacillus* has taken hold suffers from tuberculosis, but this says nothing about how that bacillus came to take hold in the patient's body i.e. the factors that combine and are sufficient, along with exposure to the bacillus, to bring about his disease.

Among modern philosophical approaches to causation, Mackie's INUS concept has been among the most helpful and was arguably the philosophical inspiration for the multicausality model

---

[50] Stehbens (1992:116).
[51] Carter (2003:201).

advocated by epidemiologists like Rothman.[52] Mackie extended Hume's idea that causes and effects are "constantly conjoined" and used the logic of necessary and sufficient conditions to describe cause and effect relations. An INUS condition is an insufficient but non-redundant part of an unnecessary but sufficient condition. In Mackie's example of a fire following a short circuit in the house wiring, the short circuit alone would not have brought about a fire but it was an essential (non-redundant) part of a set of conditions (presence of inflammable material, absence of sprinkler, etc.) that were sufficient to cause the fire.

The INUS model would be helpful for explaining cancers that can be attributed to specific pathogens as the trigger factor, for example the *helicobacter pylorus* bacterium that is associated with stomach ulcers that could develop into cancers. This bacterium is not sufficient to cause stomach cancer, nor is it necessary, as many victims show no signs of the bacterium. But clinical trials have shown that people who have it in their stomachs have significantly higher chances of contracting cancer. For those who had the bacterium and contracted stomach cancer, the presence of the bacterium would be an INUS condition which, acting together with other "unnecessary but sufficient" factors such as stress, irregular meals and ingestion of foods with high levels of carcinogens, could be a contributing cause to the patient's succumbing to cancer. In general, the presence of the bacterium would thus be viewed as raising the probability of contracting stomach cancer. This has indeed been borne out by observational clinical trials and doctors now routinely administer antibiotics to remove it when it shows up in clinical examinations.[53]

---

[52] Rothman (2002).

[53] National Cancer Institute (2013): "*Helicobacter pylori* (*H. pylori*) is a type of bacterium that is found in the stomach of about two-thirds of the world's population. *H.*

Mackie's INUS concept helped epidemiologists like Rothman and Greenland (2005) to propose multicausality models such as the "causal pie" illustrated in Fig. 2.1.

Each constellation of component causes represented in Fig.1 is minimally sufficient to produce the disease; that is, there is no redundant component cause. Each one is a necessary part of that specific causal mechanism. A specific component cause may play a role in one, two, or all three of the causal mechanisms pictured. For example, excessive gastric secretions could be the common factor 'A' in all three causal mechanisms, but the *helicobacter pylorus* is present as 'G' in the causal mechanism II. [54] A given disease can be caused by more than one causal mechanism, and every causal mechanism involves the joint action of a number of component causes.

The purpose of this brief glimpse into the philosophy of causation has been to lead us to the idea that disease causation is not

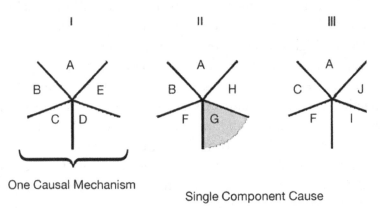

Fig. 2.1.   Causal Pie.

Source: Rothman and Greenland (2005).

---

pylori infection is a major cause of gastric (stomach) cancer and is associated with an increased risk of gastric mucosa-associated lymphoid tissue (MALT) lymphoma."

[54] This is my example. Rothman and Greenland use the example of a broken hip to make a similar point.

a simple case of discovering one or more contributing factors, and that other considerations like motivation for identifying the cause may be involved. There may also be a role for values, as discussed below. The relationship of these discussions to TCM theory will become apparent further below.

2.4 Values and Disease Causation

As a practical matter, medical scientists and researchers need to convey their findings on disease causation to health care and health policy managers who make decisions on allocation of resources to prevent and treat the disease in the communities that they manage. Multicausality models of disease are inadequate for this purpose. This may account for the appeal of the etiological standpoint to medical scientists, despite its inadequacies, as scientists need only to identify one cause for each disease and are spared the trouble of dealing with multiple and often mutually interacting causes.

With multicausality models, the scientific researcher needs to exercise judgment as to which factors to include in the causal model for statistical investigation. To the extent that values come into play in these judgments, the identification of causes is value-laden. In practice, there are numerous candidates for causal factors but, as Nagel points out, the "interest of the scientist" determines what he selects for investigation.[55] Different choices of factors lead to different causal pies.

I have used the term 'value' here in the manner that some philosophical discussions on the notion of science being value-laden have used it.[56] Some may prefer to use 'interest' instead of

---

[55] Nagel (1961: 486).
[56] See, for example, Rudner (1953) and Douglas (2009).

value, as Nagel does in the above quote. I shall continue to refer to 'value' with the caveat that it has a different meaning from its other uses such as moral values.

Take our earlier tuberculosis example. Great strides in eradicating the disease have been made since Koch's discovery of the *tubercle bacillus*, but the disease has not been stamped out. In many parts of the world, its incidence is in fact increasing with mutations to strains of the bacillus that are resistant to antibiotics (like streptomycin and rifampicin) commonly used for the treatment of the disease. The pharmacologist developing vaccines against the *tubercle bacillus* and antibiotics to kill it understandably regards the disease as being caused by a bacterium, as this would be consistent with his mission of creating agents to fight the bacillus and the value he therefore places on discovering new antibiotics. But to the epidemiologist working in poorer countries where tuberculosis is still a serious killer, the cause of tuberculosis may not be the bacillus but rather the stresses of overwork, poor diet and unhealthy sanitary conditions — these provide the basis for the bacillus to spread and take hold in the human body. Thousands in Asia and Africa die of the disease for very much the same reason that John Keats and Jane Austen are thought to have contracted the disease: poor nutrition and unhealthy living habits and conditions.

Knowledge about the kind of *tubercle bacillus* associated with fresh outbreaks of tuberculosis in some regions of the world is of limited value for controlling the spread of the disease, although it might lead to cures for those who have succumbed to it and are fortunate enough to receive treatment with antibiotics. Knowledge of the dietary factors and sanitary conditions that are associated with it, which may be obtained from epidemiological studies that include these factors in the causal pie, guides health care providers to determine optimal health expenditure plans.

Thus one can make the argument that effectiveness for achieving medical objectives would guide the researcher in the inclusion of components in the causal pie. This *"medical efficacy"* value favours research programmes that focus on causes of illness that can in practice be addressed by public health policy. A similar line of reasoning applies to TCM notions of causality in illnesses, which is focused on those factors that a person can manage in order to avoid falling ill.

2.5 Illness and its Causes in TCM Theory

We should distinguish between disease and *illness*. The term 'disease' as it is understood by Western medicine is definable as "a disorder with a specific cause (which may or may not be known) and recognisable signs and symptoms".[57] It is therefore what the doctor diagnoses the patient as having. On the other hand, as Lloyd suggests, illness is what the patient feels.[58] Illnesses therefore form a separate universe that intersects with disease. There are illnesses like the chronic fatigue syndrome that would not normally be treated as diseases. There are diseases like hepatitis B for which the carriers have the virus but do not manifest any symptoms of hepatitis and do not feel ill. The crude form of the etiological standpoint would treat all illnesses as diseases (or perhaps as chimeras, as some doctors regard chronic fatigue syndrome) although, as pointed out earlier, the etiological standpoint cannot properly incorporate illnesses for which there is no necessary or sufficient cause.

---

[57] Oxford Concised Medical Dictionary (2007).
[58] Lloyd (2003:1).

Chinese medicine, like much of ancient Greek and Galenic medicine, has traditionally been more focused on the condition of the human body when it falls ill rather than on disease and its cause. In most TCM contexts, it would be more appropriate to refer to the patient's illness than to his/her 'disease'.

TCM theory regards the fundamental factors that lead to illness as being either external climatic factors (heat, cold, dampness, wind, dryness) or internal emotions (excessive pleasure, anger, sadness, fear, and excessive contemplation) as well as accumulated products of these factors like (phlegm and blood stasis). Even though modern TCM physicians are adequately schooled in microbiological sciences and are aware of the role that viruses, bacteria and cellular disorders play in disease, this does not change their adherence to the principle that the fundamental causal factors are climatic and emotional factors and their by-products. Examples of two common diseases, the common cold and cancer, serve to illustrate this point.

2.5.1 *The common cold*

What *causes* the common cold? I once told a virologist friend that I was running a cold because I had 'caught a chill', the implication being that it was caused by a chill. He disagreed and pointed out that my cold was caused by a virus, not by a chill. When I asked where the virus had come from, he said that it was in the air and could be found everywhere. But why had I caught a cold while he had not? He thought I might have been working too hard and my immune system was down. "Since I caught the cold because my immune system was down," I argued, "and my immune system was down because I had been working too hard, would you not say that working too hard and a weakened immune system were the real causes of my cold rather than a viral infection?"

The virologist was focused on the viral etiology of the common cold while I was focused on the environmental and internal physiological factors. Both of us were guilty of what Lewis terms "invidious discrimination", each singling out a "decisive" cause of the cold and leaving the others as "causal conditions".[59] The virologist saw the rhinovirus as *the* cause of the common cold, and my weakened immune system only as a contributing condition. However, as a person interested in improving the health and fitness of people, I was biased towards the holistic picture of internal body balance and the chill that broke the back of my immune system. I saw the presence of the rhinovirus in the human body as the definition of the common cold, not its cause. As there was nothing I could do to prevent people from being exposed to that virus, my value of medical efficacy led me to look for causes that I could manage or manipulate. My search for prevention of colds would thus focus not on the virus but on dietary, exercise and hygiene factors that could be managed. The clinical trials that I would advocate for the study of causation of cold would therefore involve these causal factors.

2.5.2 *Cancer*

No other life-threatening disease is as common and causally complex as cancer. Some cancers are associated with specific pathogens, such as the *human papillomavirus* (HPV) for cervical cancer, the *helicobacter pylorus* for stomach cancer and the Hepatitis B virus for liver cirrhosis, a fatal form of liver cancer. Other cancers are associated with living habits (smoking with lung and pancreatic cancers), and still others with environmental pollutants (insecticides with nasal-pharynx cancer). There is also

---

[59] Lewis (1973:556–567).

mounting evidence that genetic factors (as in breast cancer), emotional stress (lymphoma) and high-fat diets (prostate cancer) exert significant influence.

The interpretation of statistical evidence for the impact of these varied factors on developing a malignant tumour is a treacherous enterprise as these factors exist together with a host of others that are potentially relevant. Setting up any kind of clinical trial to identify principal causal agents for specific kinds of cancer inevitably involves value judgments that determine the choice of factors to be included in the study. Such value judgments would be influenced by considerations of medical efficacy — that is, by the judgment that in a given set of social and geographical environment, those causal factors that are controllable.

This seems evident in the much-cited epidemiological study published by nutritional scientist Colin Campbell (2004) at Cornell. Based on a 20-year epidemiological investigation of a large number of population samples in various regions of China, the study concluded that a high animal protein diet (which includes dairy products, meat and fish) was the most important cause of many forms of cancer, as well as of cardiovascular disease and diabetes. Population samples in poorer parts of China that had very little animal protein in their diets showed low levels of certain cancers, even when people were exposed to higher levels of carcinogens compared with those from other regions with high animal protein diets. For example, it was found that children fed on peanuts contaminated with the fungal product *aflatoxin*, associated with liver cancer, showed lower incidence of liver cancer if they came from regions where little animal protein or dairy products was consumed.[60] As peanuts are an important

---

[60] Campbell and Campbell (2004:34–36).

source of protein and carbohydrates, and as the prevention of fungus moulds forming on peanuts requires impractical amounts of refrigeration and storage facilities, the more effective alternative would be to discourage consumption of peanuts among populations with high levels of animal protein in their diet, or to discourage the consumption of animal proteins. From this point of view, the principal cause of liver cancer in children is a diet rich in animal proteins.

In using the methods of science to investigate the causes of disease, biomedical science is influenced by the values (interests) of the medical researcher and policy makers who seek the optimal use of economic resources to achieve the objectives of health policy. That theory choice in medicine is value-laden, as some have argued it is in science, applies equally to TCM.

Chinese medicine emphasises the building up resistance to illness, as pointed out in the aphorism '*zheng qi cun nei, xie bu ke gan*' 正气存内，邪不可干 (If the body is rich in healthy *qi*, it will not succumb to external pathogens). In TCM terms, it would make more sense to regard the presence of the rhinovirus in the body as the definition of a cold rather than its cause. From the viewpoint of preventing colds, it is more useful to say that a cold is caused by exposure to weather and a weakened body defence system, because you can do something about those but very little about rhinoviruses in the air. Alternatively, taking the causal pie approach, to emphasise the segments of the causal pie relating to climatic and lifestyle factors would be more pragmatic and value-driven.

Likewise, from the TCM viewpoint, excessive emotion and inappropriate diet and living habits are the root causes of cancer rather than unusual cell growth and the rapid multiplication of cancer cells. The latter describes the mechanism by which cancers grow and take root but not the conditions that caused the cells to behave in this abnormal manner. From a biomedical viewpoint the conditions that lead to higher incidence of cancer are carcinogens, genetic factors and stress. These in turn can be related to diet, living habits and emotions, pointing to an intersection of TCM and biomedical theories of cancer causation.[61]

[61] Yu and Hong (2012) document Chinese medical explanations of the causes of various forms of cancer.

Chapter 3

Translating Chinese Medical Terms

Perhaps the best solution [to the translation problem] *will always be to refrain from seeking exact equivalents, in the case of Asian languages to coin new words from familiar roots.*

Joseph Needham

When comparing the theories of Chinese and Western medicines, another historically important issue is that of translating Chinese medical terms. This presents technical as well as ideological problems as the choice of translation is inevitably affected by the view that one takes of the scientific nature of Chinese medical concepts. The issues of translation thus lie at the heart of the difficulties in understanding and interpreting TCM theory within the framework of modern science and Western medicine.

The translation to another language of ancient technical terms used in science and medicine presents special problems because many ancient concepts do not exist in modern theories. In the case of TCM, which provides public health care to a significant proportion of Chinese nationals and is also an important alternative medical system in many East Asian countries, the problem also has political and ideological dimensions.

3.1 Historical Controversies

The translation of Chinese medical terms has a long history. The first original Chinese text to appear in a European language was a translation of the *MaiJue* ('Secrets of the Pulse') published in French in 1671.[62] In the 18th and 19th centuries, descriptions of Chinese medicine continued to reach Europe, read by scholars who might not necessarily have taken the translated terms at face value and would have delved further into their original meanings. However, with the transmission of TCM to the West as alternative medicine and the training of Western practitioners through translated texts, translation became a professional medical issue.

A study of two controversies over the correct approach to translating Chinese medical terms may be instructive towards understanding the problems of interpreting Chinese medical concepts in biomedical terms. In describing and analysing these controversies below, I have to make reference to TCM terms like 'heat', 'fire', 'organs' and 'syndromes' that have meanings different from those in ordinary language or the Western medical context. These terms will be explained in the next two chapters, and the reader's indulgence is requested at this stage to focus on the issues of translation rather than on the specific meaning of these terms.

3.1.1 *The Needham–Porkert controversy*

This controversy erupted in 1975 with the review by Needham and Lu (hereafter "Needham") of Porkert's innovative work, *The Foundations of Traditional Chinese Medicine*.[63] The reviewers dismissed Porkert's attempt to create a whole new Western

---

[62] See Wiseman (2000:180).
[63] Needham and Lu (1975); Porkert (1974).

vocabulary for Chinese medical terms, calling it a "courageous" but failed effort.

Porkert set out with the ambitious objective of providing a "methodologically adequate, coherent, and comprehensible account of the Chinese theories in a Western language [with] consistent use of a precise Western terminology to stand for that of the Chinese authors." He described his methodology as a "normative" translation approach in the sense that "a given term of the foreign language is always rendered by one and the same word (or the same few words) of our language".[64] Porkert appeared to be trying to construct a new Western vocabulary based on a scientific understanding of the concepts represented by the Chinese medical terms. The technical terms that he introduced had a distinct Western medical flavour, complete with Latin roots, such as "orb" for *zang* 藏 (organs); "orbisiconography" for *zangxiang* 藏象 (organ systems).

Particularly interesting was his translation of a key term in Chinese medicine, *qi* 气 (or 'ch'i' in the Giles–Wade system of spelling.)[65] Based on lay language equivalents used in popular books, *qi* would be "vital energy".[66] Porkert translated it as "configurational energy" and recorded 32 epithets of *qi* that are of greatest medical importance, such as *qi orthopathicum* for the Chinese term *zheng-qi* 正气, the basic "energetic resources for maintenance of physiological harmony", and *qi genuinum* for *zong-qi* 宗气 that resides in the thoracic region that controls respiration and voice.[67]

---

[64] Porkert (1974:5–7).

[65] Porkert and Needham use the old Giles–Wade spelling; as mentioned in the Preface, this book uses the modern *pinyin* system throughout, even in quotations from authors using the old system.

[66] See Reid (2001).

[67] Porkert (1974:166–173).

Underlying these translations was the interpretation of *qi* as energy of one sort or another. This does not accord with the rich mosaic of meanings that the term carries in different contexts. In one Chinese scholarly study, it has been pointed out that in the *Neijing* alone, there are over 1,700 mentions of the term *qi* with slightly different usages.[68] Most things that appeared formless were regarded as some kind of *qi*, hence the rich use of *qi* for various aspects of the human body was inevitable, for example *xieqi* 邪气 (pathogenic factors), *weiqi* 卫气 (defensive *qi* residing at the surface levels of the body) and *yingqi* 营气 (nourishing *qi* that moves through blood and organs for nourishment). Physiologically, *qi* in each of these contexts has a different meaning and function but these are related like members of a family as in Wittgenstein's family resemblances.[69]

Most Western translators, cognisant of the rich and wide usage of the word *qi*, settled for using the transliteration '*qi*' centuries ago instead of trying to find equivalents for them from Western science and medicine. Porkert may have been seeking to dispel the ambiguities of *qi* by specific categorisation into energy forms, thus taking a distinctly Western scientific interpretation of Chinese philosophy. Needham took the view that there were no equivalent words in the West for most key ancient Chinese medical terms. Adopting terms of modern science or medicine as their equivalents would in Needham's view almost certainly be wrong or misleading, distorting the thinking or the ancients: "This was precisely the great danger to which Porkert is exposing himself to with his induction and energy models".[70]

Needham objected to Porkert's invention of a series of terms not found in previous TCM literature, preferring instead the

---

[68] Wang (2001).
[69] Wittgenstein (1953:IX).
[70] Needham and Lu (1975:498).

simple literal translations of those terms complete with their ambiguities, as it was precisely because of these ambiguities that there had been "voluminous commentaries" on the medical classics through the ages.[71] For example, Porkert used "sinarteries" ('Chinese arteries') for *jingluo* 经络 (meridians) used in acupuncture. In their celebrated work on acupuncture *Celestial Lancelets*, Lu and Needham (1980) used the more ambivalent term "tracts" for *jingluo*, leaving open the question of whether these were material conduits or fixed lines like meridians in the human body.

Needham and Lu conjectured that terms used in natural and medical philosophy contained "an irreducible residue of ambiguity" and questioned the feasibility of "rendering ancient and medieval technical terms from their original languages into those understood by people living in the world of modern science and technology". At same time, they proposed a fresh approach, to create a vocabulary from semantic roots understood by international Western readers:

> It could be that in the philosophy of science there is simply no way of incorporating earlier conceptual 'paradigms' in terms of later ones ... Perhaps the best solution will always be to refrain from seeking exact equivalents, in the case of Asian languages to coin new words from familiar roots when necessary.[72]

In a rejoinder, Porkert branded Needham as a historian of science and medicine whose prime concern was "the plausibility and readability of his findings" rather than "the methodology of Chinese science in general and Chinese medicine in particular."[73] Porkert's approach was normative in the sense of translating

---

[71] Needham and Lu (1975:499).
[72] Needham and Lu (1975:491, 500).
[73] Porkert (1974:502).

Chinese medical concepts in a way that he thought would help people use TCM to diagnose and treat illnesses. We find a similar divide in the debate three decades later between Wiseman and Xie.

3.1.2 *The Wiseman–Xie debate*

This debate began when the second edition of Wiseman and Feng's *A Practical Dictionary of Chinese Medical Terms* (2002) published in China received an unfavourable review from Western medical scholar Xie Zhufan at Peking University. He disagreed with Wiseman's translation-approach based on faithfulness of translated terms to their original intended meanings in ancient Chinese medical classics.[74]

The controversy culminated in a meeting of the Western region of the World Health Organisation (WHO), at which terminological issues were debated amongst specialists from China, Korea and Japan among others. Wiseman, who wrote his PhD dissertation at Exeter on the translation of Chinese medical terms and taught medical translation at the Chang Gung University Medical faculty in Taiwan, shared with me an interesting insider perspective of the process for compiling the WHO list when I met him some years later.[75] Choosing the translations for many medical terms was apparently the subject of intense lobbying not only among the Chinese, but also Korean and Japanese specialists, for whom certain English equivalents carried different, sometimes negative, nuances in their own countries. The translation decision for each term was laboriously taken by majority vote. The final list was then

---

[74] Xie and White (2005).
[75] At Chang Geng University, Taiyuan (Taiwan) in December 2008 where he was teaching medical translation to students in TCM.

not likely to produce methodological consistency, although in the main it represented a victory for the Xie Zhufan group which had advocated extensive use of equivalent Western medical terms. The *English Translation of Common Terms in Traditional Chinese Medicine* (2004) was subsequently published with the endorsement of the Chinese Academy of Sciences and the WHO Regional Office for the Western Pacific.

Wiseman and Feng's starting point for the compilation of *A Practical Dictionary of Chinese Medicine* was "the accurate transmission of original Chinese medical knowledge", rejecting Xie's argument that "a pre-modern medicine of a distant culture must undergo adaptation before it can be of use to modern Western society". They rejected term translations that introduced Western medical connotations and terms that might "invite interference of ideas alien to Chinese medicine".[76] This ideological stance may have echoed the resentment of conservative Chinese physicians towards the encroachment by Western medicine into their medical practices through the integration policies started by Mao in the 1960s. Insistence that translation of technical terms be faithful to the original intent of the ancients amounted to rejection of efforts by modern Chinese scientists to find biomedical equivalents for the Chinese concepts, an approach thought necessary to integrate Chinese and Western medicine. By advocating a "source-oriented approach", which he deemed necessary for dealing with the "fuzziness" of Chinese medical concepts, Wiseman opted for faithfulness to the concepts of the ancient culture.[77]

The most direct form of source-oriented translations is the loanword, a word adopted from a foreign language with little or

---

[76] Wiseman and Feng (2002:17, 21).
[77] Wiseman (2000:1).

no modification.[78] For example '*mucus*' in Latin is translated as 'mucus' in English, and '*os sphenoideum*' as 'sphenoid bone'. Loanwords are rarely used in translations of Chinese medical terms, the notable exceptions being *qi*, *yin* and *yang*, which have gained currency and found their way into English dictionaries. Another form of source-oriented translations is the loan translation, which is an expression adopted from another language in a literally translated form, for example *mucus* in Latin translates to *schleim* ('slime') in German.

Xie's approach was radically different:

> Expressions proposed as the standard were carefully examined from the viewpoint of Western medicine … the proposed standard terminology had to meet the basic requirements of scientific nomenclature.[79]

Xie set himself a daunting task, insisting that such nomenclature could be established only if they "precisely reflect these concepts of Chinese medicine and at the same time are widely accepted through common practice".[80] To precisely reflect the concepts of Chinese medicine with Western words seemed to be difficult enough (in fact, as I shall argue in later chapters, it is an impossible task) without insisting that they already have wide acceptance through common practice. This courageous attempt is reminiscent of Porkert's efforts, although this time it has the virtue of not creating awkward new vocabulary but using terms already familiar in clinical work. The difficulty lies in constantly making mental adjustments and understanding

---

[78] It is similar to the transliteration, using "the closest corresponding letters of a different alphabet or language" (Oxford Concise Medical Dictionary). For Chinese translations to English, the result is generally the same as the loanword.

[79] Han in Foreword to Xie's *On Standard TCM Nomenclature* (2003).

[80] Xie (2003:1).

those familiar terms in quite different ways when they appear in Chinese medical contexts. For example, as we shall discuss in Chapter 5, 'spleen' as used in TCM has a different meaning from that of the same term in Western medicine: In TCM, it incorporates a family of functions largely to do with digestion, whereas in Western medicine the spleen removes worn-out red blood cells and other foreign bodies from the bloodstream and also serves as a reservoir of blood.

Xie's attack on the use of loan translations began with a condescending remark:

> Mr Wiseman believes that Western medical terms chosen as equivalents of Chinese medical terms should be words known to all speakers and not requiring any specialist knowledge or instrumentation (*sic*) to understand or identify, and strictly Western medical terms should be avoided … The English terms thus created … make (*sic*) the English glossary in chaos … traditional Chinese medicine is not regarded as a system of medicine but merely some Oriental folklore.[81]

Wiseman retorted that Xie's approach to translation degraded Chinese medicine:

> Biomedicised translation of Chinese medicine destroys the integrity and independence of Chinese medical concepts; it devalues Chinese medicine. It also reflects a deep-seated sense of inferiority about Chinese medicine.[82]

The reference to an inferiority complex about Chinese medicine would have touched a raw nerve in doctors like Xie who were trained in Western medicine before being required by the

---

[81] Xie *et al.* (2005:Abstract).
[82] Wiseman (2006:225).

state to study Chinese medicine with the aim of integrating it with Western medicine. They would have found assimilation of TCM by Western medicine more palatable than integration with it. At the same time they were viewed by the traditional Chinese medical community as betraying Chinese culture, submitting it to foreign domination because they suffered from an inferiority complex about the backwardness of Chinese science.

Wiseman made a strong point with his example of the term *feng huo yan* 风火眼, translated by him as "wind-fire eye", a red-eye symptom caused by a number of possible conditions, among which is having one drink too many. In TCM terminology, alcohol stokes 'fire' in the liver and mobilises 'wind' upwards to inflame the eyes. Xie's translation 'acute conjunctivitis' sounded silly to the TCM physician as a red eye normally affects more than just the conjunctiva and is not necessarily associated with an infection or with allergy as is the case with acute conjunctivitis.[83] This example indicates that Wiseman may be right to reject Western medical translations when these are clinically inaccurate. But it is does not necessarily support his more dubious (dogmatic) ideological position that being faithful to the ancients and not admitting modern biomedical interpretations of Chinese concepts make for more useful translations of Chinese medical texts.

3.2 Analysis of the Controversies

Needham's starting point was that translations should faithfully reflect the thinking of the authors of the Chinese medical classics, but this was not Porkert's primary objective. As pointed out in the last chapter, there is a clear difference between these classics

---

[83] *Taber's Cyclopaedic Medical Dictionary* (2001) lists 17 medical uses of the term conjunctivitis for inflammations of the conjunctiva.

and modern texts used in the instruction of students of TCM in China. This drove different approaches to translation, depending on whether the intention was one of medical anthropology, to reflect the original thinking of ancients, or to communicate TCM theory incorporating modern uses of these concepts that may have evolved since the ancient texts were written.

If indeed Chinese technical terms have inherent ambiguities within the Western conceptual framework, as Needham claimed, then his proposal to create new words seems like a tall order: how does one create words to fit concepts that are ambiguous? To preserve the thinking of the ancients is perhaps to make a case for the use of literal translations and to reject translations to Western medical equivalents based on modern interpretations. This would emerge later as a central issue in the debate between Wiseman and others on the use of 'source-oriented' translations.

Like the Needham–Porkert controversy, an underlying problem of the Wiseman–Xie debate is the failure of both to differentiate between translations of ancient texts and translations of technical terms used in modern texts of Chinese medicine. Wiseman's case for source-oriented translations would appear to be a strong one for scholarly translations of ancient medical classics with a view to understanding the thinking of the ancients. It has the support of German sinologist and translator of ancient Chinese medical texts, Unschuld, who argues that even though Chinese terms have different meanings when used in a Western medical context, they should have the same translations simply because

> the conceptual interpretation of reality cannot be part of the translation of the generic term employed to designate this reality; otherwise, a translation would become unfeasible (*sic*), if not impossible.[84]

---

[84] Unschuld (1989:100–102).

For example, the term *xue* 血 (blood) in the classics has some functions not found in Western medical understanding of the term, *xue* should still be translated as "blood". Unschuld seems to be simply saying that such translations are not always very good, sometimes even silly, but they are the best available.

On the other hand, modern textbooks in China were written to systematise the theory and practice of Chinese medicine and to ensure a level of uniformity in terminology for the teaching of TCM in colleges. Key portions of ancient texts like *Huangdi Neijing* as well as later works by famous physicians like Zhang Zhongjing and Li Dongyuan were extracted and subjected to interpretations with fewer ambiguities than in the original. Preservation of the thinking of the ancients was already compromised by extraction and explanation in modern language. Even the vocabulary and concepts of Western medicine crept into the terminologies used in these modern texts.

The extent to which Western medical terms could be used as equivalents of Chinese medical terms ultimately has to be limited by the differences in the theoretical foundations of the two systems of medicine. For example, Chinese diagnosis revolves around '*zheng*' 证 ('syndromes') as distinct from Western medical 'diseases'. Syndromes in TCM theory are imbalances in the body caused by deficiencies or excesses in *yin* or *yang*, or by stagnation of blood or *qi*. A TCM condition like *bi* 痹, caused by blocked or stagnating *qi*, when translated as 'arthralgia' would fail to include the variety of symptoms associated with the condition of *bi*. Arthralgia in Western medicine is severe pain in a joint,[85] and does not capture pain in the muscles and tissues nearer the skin, which *bi* includes. Wiseman uses the term 'impediment', but this is not satisfactory either as impediment

---

[85] Oxford Concise Medical Dictionary (2007).

refers to the blockage of *qi,* whereas *bi* is the resultant painful condition felt by the patient.

More extensive use of loanwords can go some way avoid such problems.[86] For example, *pi* 脾 (spleen) should be translated as the loanword *pi* when it refers to the functional system involved in digestion, which is what it principally means in TCM theory. A number of loanwords like *qi, yin* and *yang* have already entered English vocabulary through long usage. For students of TCM in English to assimilate into their vocabulary a core number of loanwords for key Chinese medical concepts would not be unreasonable to ask of people who intend to practice TCM, or of the serious reader of Chinese medical literature. With an expanded Chinese vocabulary among foreign readers of TCM texts in translation, there would be less need either to use inappropriate Western medical 'equivalents' or to live exclusively with source-oriented translations that unnecessarily retain the deep ambiguities of the ancients.

---

[86] See Buck (2000).

Chapter 4

TCM Theory: Basic Entities

If there is adequate zheng-qi, the body would not succumb
to a pathogenic attack.

Huangdi Neijing

TCM theory is built on a number of basic entities in the body and their mutual relationships that determine health, illness and the choice of therapies. These basic entities comprise *qi*, blood and body fluids essential to the functioning of the body[87] and, when the body is ill, certain pathogens like heat, phlegm and wind as well.

We begin by describing these entities as they are presented in Chinese medical textbooks before providing interpretations of the meanings and epistemic status of these entities. The objective here is not to give a comprehensive account of entities in TCM theory but rather to identify and discuss epistemological questions concerning their functions and existence and to provide biomedical interpretations of these entities to the extent that this is possible. Their descriptions in Chinese medical texts use terms and concepts that are part of TCM vocabulary and may not

---

[87] Another substance, *jing* 精 or essence, has a close relationship with *qi*. *Qi* and *jing* transform into each other, and *jing* can be interpreted as a primordial source of *qi*, while *qi*, as a form of energy, can be converted to *jing* in substantial form. *Jing* as a substance stored in the kidney and other organs will be discussed in Chapter 5.

always have equivalents in biomedical science. However it is necessary to lay out these textbook descriptions before attempting to interpret them and delve into scientific questions regarding their real existence and measurable properties.

Three of these entities — *qi*, phlegm and wind — will be analysed in more detail as each illustrates in a special way the TCM conceptual framework for physiological processes in the body.

As an exposition of TCM entities progresses, the scientist and modern physiologist usually begins to feel uncomfortable if not outraged as he is dragged from his comfort zone of cells, genes and electrochemical processes to the murkier world of abstract-like entities that he cannot see or measure. Patience and willingness toward lateral thinking will be rewarded. However, to give a foretaste of later chapters, it should be pointed out that vital organs in TCM are *clusters of functions* and not the somatic structures to which modern Western anatomy gives the same name. This in part reflects the influence of ancient Chinese thought which emphasises functions and processes rather than the physical nature of the entities involved in these functions and processes. Thus the kidney in TCM theory is not one of the two physical structures shaped like cashew nuts in the lower abdomen, but the representation of functions ranging from growth and reproduction to the processing of liquid excretion.

This apparent disregard for ontology is encountered frequently in TCM theory; in particular, in Chapter 6 when we shall see *yin* and *yang* being treated sometimes as attributes and at other times as substances.

4.1 *Qi*, Blood and Body Fluids

Although we have referred to *qi* as a substance, the physical nature that TCM attributes to it is somewhat more ambiguous.

In TCM theory, *qi* (气) has a number of specific meanings depending on the context, although most of these meanings involve a driving force behind virtually every physiological process in the body. However, when *qi* is stored in the vital organs, it is a fuel-like substance waiting to be converted to energy.

The concept of *qi* also appears in the literature on the Chinese martial arts and the *qigong* art of healing. Practitioners of these arts claim to be able to transfer some kind of life force to another person for tonic and healing purposes; they also call this *qi*. TCM theory is silent on whether such transfers are in fact possible. Whatever gets transferred by healers, if anything, may not lie within the range of meanings of *qi* with which TCM theory deals.

Blood (*xue* 血) in TCM is functionally similar to blood in Western medicine. It is closely related to *qi*. Blood flow in the body is thought to be propelled by the *qi* of the heart. If this heart-*qi* is inadequate, blood would become too weak to circulate and this can have an impact on the working of the mind, causing conditions such as restlessness and insomnia. Other internal organs like the lung, spleen and liver are also involved in the movement of blood. The lung is thought to be connected to all vessels of the body (hence the aphorism 'the lung is connected to all vessels' *fei chao baimai* 肺朝百脉); it accumulates *qi* and blood from the whole body to assist the heart in propelling blood movement in the body. The spleen is said to 'command' blood, directing it to circulate normally and preventing it from flowing out of the blood vessels. The liver stores blood and regulates the volume of blood, smoothing the activity of *qi* to promote blood circulation.

Factors that can affect blood circulation are the state of the vessels and the changes of the body's internal environment expressed in TCM terms like cold, heat, phlegm, dampness, blood stasis, as well as swellings and nodules.

Blood and *qi* are so closely related that they behave somewhat like two sides of the same coin. TCM theory puts it this way: 'Blood is the mother of *qi* and *qi* is the marshal of blood (血为气之母，气为血之帅).' Blood carries *qi* and is also essential to the production of *qi* by providing nutrients to the vital organs and the meridians. *Qi* is the driving force that enables blood circulation; as we noted earlier, *qi* also plays a role in the production of blood.

Body fluids (*jinye* 津液) help maintain life activities in the body. Body fluids contain mainly water and nutrients. They are components of fluid in the blood vessels and also flow outside the vessels in the vital organs. Body fluids can be excreted as tears, nasal discharges and saliva. Moistening and nourishing, as well as the transportation of used (turbid) *qi* for excretion are key functions of body fluids.

By assigning a variety of functions to each of the three basic substances *qi*, blood and body fluids, TCM theory tries to capture all the known and observable physiological processes in the body that involve the movement of these substances up and down and around the body, and from the inside to the outside of the body.

4.2 Pathogens

Besides the essential entities of *qi*, blood and body fluids in the body, illness-causing pathogens of various kinds may reside in the body. These are classified as either *exogenous* pathogens, originating from climatic factors outside the body, or *endogenous* pathogens that are created within the body.

Endogenous pathogens used in its wider sense refer to primary internal factors that cause organs to be dysfunctional, leading to illness. The term covers five pathogenic factors whose behaviours have similarities to those of external climatic pathogenic factors, namely wind (*feng* 风), cold, dampness, dryness and heat.[88] Phlegm (*tan* 痰) and blood stasis (*yuxue* 瘀血) are regarded as secondary endogenous pathogens as they are pathological substances created by endogenous factors. We briefly describe these latter pathogens below. (The "seven emotions", which will be dealt with in Chapter 6, are sometimes also regarded as endogenous pathogens as they can also impair organ function and physiological processes.)

Descriptions of pathogens draw on the concept pairs of *yin-yang* and deficiency-excess. *Yin* and *yang* are opposing characteristics. *Yin* is soft, dark and cool, whilst *yang* is hard, bright and warm. Deficiency and excess are also referred to as asthenic and sthenic conditions, and these are the rough equivalents of depletion and repletion respectively in ancient Greco-Roman medicine. Deficiency is usually characterised by inadequacy of energy and paleness of complexion, excess by restlessness and a reddish complexion. (Deficiency and excess will be discussed further in Chapter 6 under *syndromes*.)

4.2.1 *Wind*

Wind that is part of the external climatic environment is *exogenous wind*; it is considered a vile source of illness as it is thought to penetrate the skin and bring about a variety of conditions such as headache, joint stiffness and arthritic pain. In combination with cold, heat or dampness, it can lead to sore throats, coughs and colds and fevers. A characteristic of ailments caused by exogenous

---

[88] Wu (2002:161–162) describes "the five endogenous pathogenic factors" (*neisheng wuxie* 内生五邪); Chai (2007) refers to all internal factors collectively as endogenous pathogens (*neishang bingyin* 内伤病因).

wind is movement; hence arthritic pain that moves from one part of the body to another is thought to involve the wind pathogen.

Endogenous wind, because it is characterised by movement, may be regarded as an extension of the exogenous wind concept to processes inside the body. In TCM theory, endogenous wind is produced by pathological processes in the liver. It is usually referred to as 'liver-wind' and its movement as 'internal disturbance of liver-wind' (*ganfeng neidong* 肝风内动).

As we shall see below, the connection between exogenous wind and endogenous wind is quite tenuous, having in common mainly the tendency to move from one part of the body to another. Attempts beyond this etymological explanation to attribute a common physiological basis for TCM wind may not therefore be very useful.

4.2.2 *Cold and heat*

Endogenous cold arises from deficiency in *yang*. As the kidney *yang* is the source of warming of the whole body, deficiency in kidney *yang* is the predominant contributor to endogenous cold. Endogenous heat, on the other hand, comes from a variety of sources, including emotional stresses, deficiency of *yin* (causing *yang* to be dominant), and exogenous wind and cold that transform into heat.[89]

4.2.3 *Dampness and dryness*

Endogenous dampness is thought to arise from the spleen which in TCM theory has the function of transforming water into *qi* as part of the digestive process in the body. Dysfunction of the spleen causes fluid to accumulate and disrupt the spleen's 'food-transforming and transportation' function; it can also produce

---

[89] Heat and cold will be further discussed under *syndromes* in Chapter 6.

phlegm. Endogenous dryness is associated with deficiency of *yin* and/or blood, and is manifested in the observable dryness of the eyes, nose and throat, as well as (by the TCM conceptual framework) in the intestines, lung and stomach where it is not observable except by its supposed manifestations.

4.2.4 *Phlegm*

Phlegm in TCM refers not just to sputum, the sticky viscous substance that lines one's throat and bronchioles, causing irritation and coughing as the body tries to expel it. Phlegm in TCM also takes the form of nasty clear fluids that inhabit the vital organs, causing ailments ranging from indigestion, lassitude, insomnia and irascible moods to headaches, epilepsy and strokes, earning it the aphorism 'a hundred ailments are induced by phlegm' (*baibing duoyou tan zuosui* 百病多由痰作祟) and 'strange diseases are caused mainly by phlegm' (*guaibing duo tan* 怪病多痰).

4.2.5 *Blood stasis*

Blood stasis (*yuxue* 瘀血) in TCM is a pathological substance, a by-product of disturbances in blood circulation, leading to clots, subcutaneous purpura or lumps. When stasis is not manifested in clots or lumps but is more widespread, it is thought to cause general pain, irregular pulse and manic anxiety. It is caused by exogenous climatic factors like the cold that causes blood to stagnate or coagulate, or by emotional factors. The condition or pathological process that leads to the formation of blood stasis is termed 'blood stagnation' (*xueye* 血瘀) in TCM. It is thought to be caused by exogenous factors such as prolonged exposure to the cold and by certain emotions that upset internal balance.

As most TCM entities are complex and have multifarious meanings depending on the context of their use, and as many aspects of each of these entities are unobservable (in a sense similar to that of electrons not being directly observable whilst cells, genes and neurotransmitters are), the familiar question arises as to the supposed ontological status of these concepts and entities. We address this key question now by a more detailed analysis of three entities: *qi*, phlegm and wind.

Having outlined the TCM textbook presentation of these basic entities, we now address the more challenging issue of how to interpret the meaning of these entities and their relevance to the physiology of health and illness.

4.3 Understanding *Qi* (气)

Qi is undoubtedly the central and the most pervasive entity in TCM theory. In ancient Chinese cosmology, *qi* was the primordial ether-like substance that constituted the universe at the beginning of time. It transformed into all the substances in the universe and also became the moving force behind all physical processes, including physiological processes in living things. In the Chinese language, the word *qi* is to be found as a component of hundreds of compound words whose meanings cover almost every aspect of the universe, from the weather (*qixiang* 气象) and evil forces (*xieqi* 邪气) to the glow of health on one's face (*qise* 气色) and the spirit of an artistic work (*qiyun* 气韵).

In distant antiquity, concepts of *qi* from philosophy found their way into the theory of Chinese medicine, which came to regard *qi* as the basic constituent of the human body as well as the substance that maintains the body's life processes. Lay treatments of *qi* in popular books on TCM commonly describe it as "vital energy" while also referring to its storability as a substance within the vital organs.[90]

---

[90] Reid (2001).

In fact, ancient Chinese thought did not distinguish between matter and energy. A somewhat extravagant claim could be made that the absence of a matter–energy duality reflected the deep insights of Chinese thought that presaged the discovery of mutual convertibility of matter and energy in 20th century physics. It is more likely that the Chinese, with their traditional lack of interest in ontology, simply never bothered with these ontological distinctions. This proved to be not far removed from the pathbreaking discoveries of Albert Einstein and modern physics.

Like ancient philosophy, Chinese medicine was more concerned with the functions and actions of *qi* than its intrinsic nature. Some scholars have interpreted *qi* as "matter on the verge of becoming energy, or energy at the point of materialising".[91] This appears to be deliberately vague, inspired perhaps by the Chinese Doctrine of the Golden Mean that advocates seeking a compromise between two competing claims.

Qi presents two related epistemic questions pertaining to its observability and to the possible existence of an entity underlying its multiple manifestations. Because *qi* has so many meanings even within TCM theory, questions regarding whether or not it is observable, or measurable by scientific instruments, or its effects are testable, cannot be meaningfully addressed unless we are specific about which meaning of *qi* we have in mind. A common meaning of *qi* as an observable entity is air which in TCM theory is absorbed by the lung and converted into other forms of *qi* after interacting with other substances in the body. The many other meanings of *qi* are best explained by enumerating, in accordance with TCM theory, the various physiological processes that involve *qi*. After explaining these physiological processes, I shall provide an interpretation of *qi* that eschews the

---

[91] See Kaptchuk (2000:43) and the references to Sivin (1976) and Bennet (1978).

classical Chinese notion that there is a distinct entity underlying these processes.

Qi is classified into various forms in Chinese medical literature to describe specific capabilities involved in physiological processes. The classifications within the classical Chinese medical theory of *qi* are summarised below.[92]

4.3.1 *Classical Chinese medical theory of Qi*

4.3.1.1 *Formation and classification*

Various forms of *qi* are classified by origin, function and location:

By origin: *Yuan-qi* (元气), or primordial *qi*, is inherited in the first instance from parents and stored in the vital organs (mainly the 'kidney') and the meridians and collaterals. Acquired *qi*, on the other hand, is generated from air and food after birth throughout life. Part of it can be converted to replenish the body's stock of *yuan-qi* which is depleted by work, stress and illness.

By function: The main forms are pectoral-*qi*, nutrient-*qi* and defensive-*qi*. Pectoral-*qi* or *zong-qi* (宗气) is situated in the thoracic area, warming the blood vessels and nourishing the lung; an abundance of it gives a person a sonorous voice. Nutrient-*qi* or *ying-qi* (营气) circulates in the body and nourishes the internal organs. Defensive-*qi* or *wei-qi* (卫气) circulates in the outer layer of the body and forms an armour that defends against external pathogens. When it is weak, the body is vulnerable to harmful climatic influences like cold, wind, dampness and heat. Defensive *qi* also helps regulate sweat to maintain body temperature.

---

[92] Based on the *Huangdi Neijing*, two college texts on TCM theory, Wang (2001) and the entry "*Qi*" in the Encyclopedia of Chinese Medicine *Zhongguo Dabaikequanshu*.

By location: *Qi* is present in every organ and along the meridians, hence the existence of such terms as heart-*qi*, spleen-*qi*, stomach-*qi* and lung-*qi* as well as meridian *qi*. Each kind of *qi* has one or more roles related to the functions of these organs and of the meridians.

4.3.1.2 *Physiological functions of qi*

The principal functions of *qi* are as follows.

The *propelling* function that drives blood, enables fluid passage within the body, and is the moving force behind digestion.

The *warming* function, with *qi* as a source of heat for the body, carrying nourishment with it for body tissues. This function explains why an inadequate level of *qi* can be associated with cold hands and feet.

The *protective* function, with circulating *qi* at the surface level of the body and so protecting it against invasions of external pathogens such as wind and cold.

The *nutrient* function, with nutrient *qi* (*ying-qi*) derived from digestive processes being converted into material constituents of the organs and meridians, as well as providing the energy and driving force for physiological processes in the living body.[93]

The *fixating* or consolidating function, which holds back fluid to stay within blood vessels and tissues and prevents excessive loss of fluid by sweating and blood oozing out of blood vessels.

The *transforming* function, converting food into a kind of essence for nutrition, transforming one kind of fluid into another, and helping the excretion of waste substances.

The *intermediation* function, connecting and harmonising the functions of the various organs through the movements of *qi* along

---

[93] Wu (2000:43).

the meridians and collaterals, as well as up and down the trunk of the body and between the inner and outer layers of the body.[94]

These functions are reflected by the roles of *qi* in two core areas of TCM theory — in the mind-body relationship, and in pathogenesis and related therapy.

Qi's role in the mind-body relationship: The *Neijing* states that "the five zang-organs…transform five kinds of *qi* to generate the emotions of joy, anger, contemplation, anxiety and fear."[95] Each kind of *qi* activity takes place in an individual organ and produces an emotion that can in turn cause harm to the organ or another part of the body. For example, anger harms the liver, causing imbalances that result in headaches, convulsions, dizziness or strokes, or a combination of these. Likewise, excessive 'contemplation' (amounting to brooding) results in impaired spleen-*qi*, leading to disorders in digestion.[96]

Qi's role in pathogenesis and therapy: Pathogenesis refers to the origination and development of an illness. Within the framework of TCM models, this is described in terms of the origination of syndromes and the dynamics of their transformation into other syndromes as the illness progresses (see Chapter 6). Two common *qi*-related syndromes are *qi* deficiency (low level of *qi*) and obstruction in the flow of *qi*. The former could be the result of physical stress or the depletion of *qi* because of illness; the latter can be brought about by the presence of dampness and phlegm

---

[94] Wang (2001:71–72).

[95] *Yellow Emperor's Canon of Medicine* (2005:731) *Suwen, Tianyuanji Dalunpian*.

[96] "…all diseases are caused by the disorder of *qi*. For example, anger drives *qi* to flow upwards, excessive joy slackens *qi*, sorrow exhausts *qi*, fear makes the *qi* sink, and excessive contemplation binds *qi*." *Jutong Lunpian* (Discussion of Pains), 481. See Wang (2001:467–472).

in the body that impedes free *qi* movement, or by emotional factors such as anger or anxiety that cause stagnation of liver *qi*. Because of the close relationship between *qi* and blood, obstruction in *qi* flow is commonly accompanied by disorders in blood circulation such as blood stagnation.

The appropriate therapy for an existing syndrome lies in restoring balance. In our examples, this involves correcting *qi* deficiency with *qi* tonics and restoring *qi* flow with *qi*-regulating medications or acupuncture treatments.

Zheng-qi: Another common meaning of *qi* encountered in Chinese medical texts is *zheng-qi* (正气), an overarching term that encapsulates all forms of *qi* that drive the physiological processes in the body, protect it against disease-causing pathogens, and give the body the capacity to recover from illness. The function of protection against pathogens is similar to that of the immune system in Western medicine. *Zheng-qi* is translated variously as upright *qi*, true *qi*, genuine *qi*, vital *qi* and healthy *qi*.

The *Neijing*'s prescription for preventing illness is captured in the famous aphorism 'if there is adequate *zheng-qi*, the body would not succumb to a pathogenic attack' (*zheng-qi cun nei, xie bu ke gan* 正气存内，邪不可干). As *zheng-qi* is the totality of various forms of *qi* that drive the body and protect it, the *Neijing*'s medical insight lies in enjoining people to cultivate all the forms of *qi* that together constitute the body's defences against natural external pathogens as well as internal pathogens produced by bad emotions and poor living habits.

4.3.2 *Interpreting qi*

Even more meanings of *qi* than the principal ones enumerated above can be found in the literature of Chinese medicine. According to one estimate, in the medical classic *Huangdi Neijing* alone, there are 1,700 different uses of the word *qi*.[97] Questions that naturally arise include:

1. Is *qi* a substance or a form of energy?
2. What, if anything, is the commonality underlying the various meanings of *qi* in Chinese medical theory?
3. Is *qi* a real entity or a 'convenient fiction'? In other words, is the theory of *qi* meant to be interpreted realistically or is the theory to be taken as talking about merely fictional entities, introduced to codify the phenomena in a convenient way?

On the first question, as pointed out earlier, the distinction between matter and energy tends to be blurred in Chinese philosophy, and this is reflected in the TCM concept of *qi*. Where these distinctions are being made, *qi* is a substance in some of its roles and a form of energy in others.

The second question arises only because believers in conventional TCM theory presuppose that a common entity underlies all the functions that *qi* performs. This is the implicit commonly accepted understanding of physicians trained in TCM, and textbooks reflect this understanding by enumerating the various kinds of *qi* and their functions, as was done above under "The classical theory of *qi*". No common entity need exist for the classical theory of *qi* to be meaningful or useful. The commonality underlying the various meanings of *qi* in TCM theory seems to be that the notion of *qi* is invoked in descriptions of all physiological processes in the human body. Nothing moves or changes without some role played by *qi*. In effect, *qi* can be viewed as a concept that covers all change and movement. Some kind of *qi*, or a form of *qi*, is involved in moving blood and fluids, in

---

[97] Wang (2001:44).

digestion of food, in excretion of waste matter, in generating emotions originating in the organs, in the production of blood, and so on.

This view of *qi* as a generic term for the agent of change would be in line with ancient Chinese philosophy's view of the world as beginning with *qi*, which materialised into animate as well as inanimate bodies, and which also drives all processes. Considered in this light, questions regarding the observability and measurability of *qi* and its ontological status are meaningful only with reference to the specific contextual meaning of *qi*. For example, pectoral-*qi* is the kind of *qi* that is presumed by TCM theory to exist in the thoracic region, warming the blood vessels and nourishing the lung; an abundance of it gives a person a sonorous voice. Orthodox Chinese physicians faithful to ancient texts would likely be comfortable with the claim, in the manner of Maxwell (1962), that pectoral-*qi* exists in reality but science has not yet found a way of detecting and measuring it. But the modern TCM physician well-versed in anatomy and physiology might well find it more comfortable to see pectoral-*qi* as a metaphor for the ability of the lungs to do their work in assisting blood circulation and generating voice. One could take the power of a person's voice as a proxy for his level of pectoral-*qi* and set up a measurement scale based on his vocal power. Indeed the ordinary language Chinese expression for someone with a powerful voice is that he is 'abundant in pectoral-*qi*'. *Pectoral-qi* in this context would merely be a way of expressing functional aspects of the lungs and diaphragm that are involved in breathing, blood circulation and voice production. In that limited sense, it is a convenient fiction, similar to the kind that the scientific instrumentalist has in mind for entities in physics. It is a representation not necessarily of some underlying real material entity but rather of a physiological capability of the body.

What matters ultimately is whether or not there is independent evidence for the truth of those parts of TCM theory that invoke *qi*. Every observable situation involving a patient can be given a *post hoc* interpretation in terms of the TCM categories and *qi* in particular. The pertinent question is whether once thus interpreted, predictions are made that can then be tested. I shall argue in Chapter 7 that testable predictions can indeed be made.

Likewise, the concept of spleen-*qi* is an attempt to capture the capability of the body's digestive system to transform food into a form for assimilation to provide energy and repair or create new tissue. The spleen in TCM theory is the organ responsible for digestive processes. A weakness of spleen-*qi* causes poor digestion, a bloated stomach, loose stools and a weakened constitution, manifested in a weak pulse, pale tongue with whitish fur, softened voice and general lassitude. The body's digestive processes behave as if they were driven by a kind of internal vital energy (spleen-*qi*). Put in another way, to say that *qi* of the spleen is weak is another way of expressing the clinical claim that certain symptoms of digestive disorder can be alleviated by TCM interventions such as *qi* tonic herbs (for example, *Astragalus* and ginseng root). The empirical basis for such a claim must be clinical experience, and the acceptance of such a claim would be through clinical trials to show that these symptoms can be relieved by herbs classified as spleen-*qi* tonics. In sum, the starting point is empirical observation: certain herbs are found to relieve a specific set of symptoms, and an explanation was found through defining these symptoms as those of a weakened spleen-*qi* and accordingly classifying these herbs as tonics for spleen-*qi*.

4.4 Phlegm (*tan* 痰): The Ubiquitous Pathogen

Among the internal pathogens that disturb the human body, phlegm or *tan* (痰) is arguably the most troublesome. Its importance in TCM theory and clinical work rivals that of *qi*, its antithesis and nemesis.

Phlegm is a difficult concept to explain and understand even within the framework of TCM theory, according to which phlegm pervades most parts of the body and lies at the root of many internal disorders. Interestingly, what goes by the name of phlegm also played a key role in ancient Greco-Roman medicine: Galen listed it as one of the four humours alongside blood, choler and black bile, attributing one's temperament to the balance of these humours. He did not, however, give phlegm the wide and powerful influence that it finds in TCM.

In TCM theory, phlegm is generated in the internal organs as a result of the accumulation of dampness and fluids in the body. The explanation of phlegm production draws on several aspects of TCM theory, including the functions of organs (see Chapter 5). Various pathogenic factors, including climatic and emotional factors, improper diet and excessive stress, can impair the internal organs and affect the activity of *qi*, leading to disturbances in the normal movements of body fluids, the accumulation of these fluids, and the eventual production of phlegm.[98] The spleen in TCM governs transportation and transformation of water and dampness, the lung regulates water passage, the kidney governs water, the liver promotes the metabolism of body fluid, and the trunk of the body serves as the main water passage in the body.[99] A disorder of any of these organs may lead to retention of body fluids and accumulation of dampness, which turns into phlegm.

Phlegm is in fact only one of a family of four pathogens that can transform from one form to another, namely, in increasing

---

[98] See, for example, Wu (2002:173) and Wu (2000:133).
[99] The trunk of the body in TCM is deemed a hollow organ (*fu*-organ), termed *sanjiao* 三焦 or 'triple energiser'.

order of viscosity — dampness, water, rheum (*yin* 饮) and phlegm. We deal here only with phlegm, the nastiest and most ubiquitous of the quartet, as a means of highlighting an ontological aspect of TCM pathogens.

Phlegm that coagulates into solid form in the lung is observable as sputum. This process underlies the ancient saying, "The spleen is the source of phlegm and the lung is the container of phlegm."[100]

Once it takes hold, phlegm (supposedly in fluid form) can spread and inhabit nearly all parts of the body, causing a variety of troublesome conditions, including:

1. Hindrance of the flow of *qi* in the meridians and of blood throughout the body, leading to numbness, limb inflexibility, subcutaneous nodules and abscesses.
2. Obstruction of the activity of *qi* in the internal organs. For example, in the lung, this causes coughs, chest tightness and dyspnoea (difficulty in breathing); in the stomach, it is associated with nausea and vomiting.
3. Confusion of the mind when it invades parts of the body from the chest upwards. This can be associated with dizziness, delirium, chest oppression or syncope.
4. An assortment of complex symptoms, depending on where phlegm accumulates ranging from numbness and arthralgia to vomiting, dizziness, palpitations and cerebral strokes.

The physical nature of phlegm is described in TCM literature as either 'with form' or 'without form'. The former is manifested in coagulated form as sputum in the lungs and respiratory tract whilst the latter behaves like a fluid that permeates many parts of

---

[100]Wu (2002:174).

the body.[101] While phlegm in the form of sputum is easily definable and observable, its nature as a formless fluid is more obscure.
The classic description in Chinese medical literature of formless
phlegm is of a fluid that pervades many parts of a human body
suffering from its ill effects, but a modern TCM researcher would
be hard put to isolate and collect formless phlegm from a vivisec-
tion of the organs that it is deemed to inhabit. There are so many
fluids to be found in these organs that it is doubtful that any such
researcher would be able to isolate phlegm from these fluids
given that TCM theory does not define its chemical composition.
It seems that the only defensible interpretation is that it be
regarded merely as a 'fictional' proxy for the presence of certain
classical symptoms of phlegm retention.

Why did the ancients group all four of these apparently dis-
parate conditions (sets of symptoms) listed above under the category of illnesses caused by phlegm? Would it not have been
simpler to give a different name to each pathogen that caused a
different set of symptoms? My conjecture is that in the history of
clinical experimentation with herbal remedies, it was discovered
that certain herbs could be used to treat a variety of conditions.
Because the four sets of symptoms listed above enjoyed the commonality of being treatable with certain herbs, and because one set
of symptoms involves coughing out solid phlegm (sputum), they
were grouped together as illnesses caused by the presence of (solid
or formless) phlegm, and the herbs classified as phlegm-resolving
herbs. These herbs became the main ingredients of formulations
to treat this group of conditions. Each formulation would be used
to treat a different condition, like a wet cough, or convulsions and
dizziness, but *the formulation would use one or more phlegm-resolving herbs.* In other words, the different pathological conditions

---

[101]Wu (2000).

might have been grouped together because they appeared to have something in common — they enjoyed relief from certain herbs or formulations containing these herbs. An example might help to elucidate this point.

The herbs *banxia* 半夏 (*rhizoma pinellieae*) and *jupi* 橘皮 (*pericarpiun citri tangerinae*), the dried and aged peels of Chinese tangerines, have from ancient times been found to be effective in treating cough with white sputum. *Banxia* is a phlegm-resolving herb; *jupi* regulates *qi* to eliminate dampness[102]; it also helps to prevent the formation of more phlegm transformed from dampness. They are the main ingredients of the popular formulation for cough with sputum called *Erchen Tang* 二陈汤. This formulation also includes *fuling* 茯苓 (*poria*), a diuretic that complements the dampness-eliminating function of *jupi*, and *gancao* 甘草 (liquorice), for harmonising the effect of the other three herbs.

By adding two herbs to the four already in *Erchen Tang*, a different disorder could be treated, the so-called 'disharmony between gall bladder and stomach', a condition manifested in nervousness, dizziness, heart palpitations, vexation, insomnia or restless sleep with troubling dreams and, in extreme instances, epileptic fits. The formulation *Wendan Tang* 温胆汤 comprises *Erchen Tang* plus two herbs, *zhuru* 竹茹 (*caulis bambusae in taeniam*) and *zhishi* 枳实 (*fructus aurantii imaturus*). *Zhuru* clears heat, whilst *zhishi* complements the role of *jupi* in 'regulating' (assisting in the flow of) *qi* and dispersing phlegm (see Table 4.1).

The phlegm that is being combated with *Wendan Tang* is not the coagulated phlegm in the lungs that causes cough, but the formless and unobservable phlegm in the organs and the head that causes quite different symptoms like vexation, nervousness and dizziness. It is not the case that the latter symptoms are being

---

[102] The term 'regulate' (*li* 理) has a specific meaning in TCM theory. It refers to promoting flow. Hence regulating *qi* is promoting its flow in the body.

Table 4.1   Formulation of *Erchen Tang* and *Wendan Tang.*

Ingredients		Functionality
Erchen Tang	*Wendan Tang*	
Banxia	Banxia	Resolves phlegm
Jupi	Jupi	Regulates *qi* and removes dampness
Fuling	Fuling	Removes dampness
Gancao	Ganco	Harmonises the other herbs
	Zhuru	Clears internal heat
	Zhishi	Regulates *qi* and removes dampness

resolved by the other two ingredients *zhuru* and *zhishi*. Clinical experience indicates that these two herbs by themselves are not able to achieve phlegm-resolving results, unlike *banxia* which can do so even acting alone, although more effectively when combined with the other herbs. In other words, both illnesses can be treated by formulations that necessarily contain a phlegm-resolving herb, *banxia* in this example.

The explanatory burden of phlegm covers a multitude of sins. It is a proxy for those physiological factors that bring about clinical conditions classified by TCM as phlegm-related. Phlegm (except as sputum) is not directly observable because, from a biomedical standpoint, it does not exist as a substance. I interpret it as an abstraction of a number of biomedical substances in the body that work together to cause certain disorders in the body. The body suffering from the effects of phlegm behaves *as if* such some substance called phlegm was present inside. Are such abstractions either necessary or useful in TCM theory? A social science analogy might be relevant here.

Supposing there was disunity of staff in an organisation, and the management thus sets out to rectify the situation by promoting cooperation and inculcating a common sense of purpose, thereby eliminating the entity of 'disunity'. At a different time and age, spiritual diviners might have attributed the bad humour of the staff to the invasion of the evil spirit of disunity. Acting as if this spirit existed, although not observable by the common man (diviners might claim to see them), the management goes about boosting staff morale, providing financial incentives and the like, based on the advice of the diviners who gain their insights through mediation with the bad spirit and also offer prayers to placate it and make it go away. The end result is that disunity is resolved. Steps are also taken to discourage or block its return. Had modern sociological theory been applied instead, the remedy might have been very similar or the same (including the use of prayers, albeit to a different spirit). The ontological status of the disunity spirit is of little relevance to those who merely wanted to know what to do to eliminate its influence on their organisations.

Phlegm is like a bad spirit that yields mischievous influences on the body identified by classical symptoms associated with its presence. These symptoms in effect define phlegm, and could be simply be called 'phlegm symptoms' with the word 'phlegm' in adjectival form to denote the particular family of symptoms that TCM theory associates with phlegm.

TCM theory simplified the world to a limited number of pathogens; hence entities like phlegm carried the burden of blame for 'a hundred ailments' and 'strange diseases'. Herbal remedies for phlegm-based disorders were found. A variety of leaves, roots and animal parts are available that clinical experience indicates are able to help in 'phlegm elimination'. They are combined with other herbs, drawing on the method of medical formulations that consist of cocktails of herbs combined in such a way as to maximise the desired overall therapeutic effect. In such a cocktail one or more herbs play the principal ('monarch') role of directly addressing the medical condition. In the case of phlegm-related conditions, *banxia* is a commonly used principal herb, as is the case with the two formulations *Erchen Tang* and *Wendan Tang* analysed above.

4.5 Wind (*feng* 风): An Ill that Blows No Good

Exogenous wind, originating from the external environment, is thought to penetrate the skin and have the ability to move to various parts of the body and a tendency to go to the head and face, with manifestations of headache, running nose, sweating and aversion to cold. It has high mobility (as is the case with rubella which is marked by quick fluctuations in *cutaneous pruritus* or skin itch) and has no fixed location; hence the Chinese term *fengzhen* 风疹 or 'wind rash' for rubella.

Because of its propensity for movement and change, other external pathogens like dampness, cold, heat and dryness are regarded as tending to attach themselves to wind. For example, wind combined with dampness causes rheumatic conditions (*fengshi* 风湿); wind and cold bring about the wind-cold syndrome (*fenghan* 风寒) associated with colds and flu infections.

Endogenous wind in TCM theory is created internally in the body, principally in the liver. Standard explanations of how endogenous wind is produced draw on the concepts of *yin* and *yang*. When used here to explain the production of wind in the liver, *yin* and *yang* are attributes describing contrasting states of the liver. *Yin* is a physical state characterised by moistness, coolness and quietness; *yang* by dryness, heat and activity; in a healthy liver, *yin* and *yang* are in balance. TCM theory deems endogenous wind to be produced under one or more of four conditions:

(a) Extreme heat that scorches the *yin* of the liver and can lead to convulsions;
(b) The *yang* of the liver is transformed into wind, disturbing the upper orifices and causing dizziness and convulsions;

(c) The presence of *yin* deficiency causes *yang* to ascend, stirring up wind in the process and causing inadequate nourishment for the tendons and ligaments, leading to convulsions;

(d) Blood deficiency results in lack of nourishment for the liver and tendons, stirring up wind that is manifested as muscular peristalsis and tremors.

In the case of (a), when the *yin* of the liver is damaged by heat, balance is upset, *yang* gains ascendancy, becomes hyperactive and brings about convulsions. In the case of (b) and (c), *yin* and *yang* behave like substances in the liver. When the *yang* of the liver is in excess, it can be converted into wind; when there is deficiency in *yin*, *yang* becomes relatively stronger and ascends, stirring up wind in the process.

Chinese medical theory has not always drawn a firm distinction between exogenous and endogenous wind. Before the *Jin-Yuan* dynasties, exogenous wind was regarded as a cause of *zhongfeng* 中风 or cerebral strokes. Later texts attributed the condition to internal processes that are now described as by TCM theory as endogenous wind.[103] There does not appear to be any direction relation between exogenous and endogenous wind.[104] Symptoms of conditions associated with wind of either kind have some similarities such as the tendency to move its locus (from skin to meridians, from liver to head and orifices, etc.), but the similarity ends there. Yet exogenous and endogenous winds are treated as though they were the same entity manifesting itself in different situations and locations. There is no basis for treating them as manifestations of the same underlying biochemical

---

[103] Wang (2001:455).

[104] If a body deficient in *qi* suffers an attack of exogenous wind when there is a sudden change in weather, it can trigger reactions that eventually lead to the formation of endogenous wind. See Zhou (2007), 303.

entity, and the explanation for TCM theory's use of the term to describe quite different physiological phenomena must be sought elsewhere. A biomedical interpretation of wind would indeed be an interesting area for clinical research.

Unlike phlegm, which is understood by TCM theory to be a substance that can at least sometimes be manifested externally — as solid sputum in the lungs, the ontological status of wind is even more ambiguous. External atmospheric wind is considered to have penetrated the body's surface to bring about symptoms like a running nose and aching joints, whilst endogenous wind is thought to move from liver to head to cause dizziness and convulsions. But a modern TCM physician would be under no illusion that there are breezes blowing in aching joints and ligaments or, in the case of endogenous wind, gaseous movement in the head. Like phlegm, wind is a ghost entity that is used to conveniently explain physiological symptoms in the body marked by movement and changeability.

As was the case for phlegm described earlier, there are herbs that have been found to relieve conditions with symptoms of wind, be it endogenous or exogenous wind. This may historically have lent strength to the idea that a basic entity wind is the common factor behind these conditions. For example, the herb *fangfeng* 防风 (*radix saposhnikoviae*) literally means 'resisting wind'. It is used to relieve 'exogenous wind symptoms' like headaches and arthritic pains of wind-dampness. But it has also been used to treat ailments like infantile convulsions attributed to endogenous wind. Since exogenous wind is readily observable, *fangfeng* is likely to have been discovered first for treating symptoms thought to be caused by exogenous wind. Later when it was also found to relieve symptoms like a form of arthritis in which pains are not fixed in one part of the body but move from one place to another, mimicking the movements of wind, the arthritis would have been attributed to endogenous wind. Recent clinical research has indicated that *fangfeng* contains anti-spasmodic ingredients that could play a calming role in conditions like headache, intestinal irritability and convulsions, all of which are often accompanied by muscular spasms. Thus wind in TCM could well be a proxy for a family of conditions in which muscular spasms are present.

Another common herb used to treat wind is *tianma* 天麻 (*rhizoma gastrodiae*) of the orchid family. *Tianma* however is used for treating only endogenous wind, to "arrest convulsions, calm the liver and suppress (an exuberant) *yang*".[105] Combined with other herbs, it is used to treat conditions varying from convulsions and dizziness to tension headaches and hypertension. For example, the decoction *Tianma Gouteng Yin* 天麻钩藤饮, commonly used for certain types of hypertensive condition, comprises 10 herbs, with *tianma* and another herb *gouteng* (*ramulus uncariae cum uncis*) used commonly to treat 'endogenous wind', playing the monarch roles in the formulation. This decoction also contains *zhizi* 栀子 (*fructus gardeniae) and huangqin* 黄芩 (*radix scutellariae*) which have the functions of clearing excess heat in the liver meridian. With endogenous wind as the primary underlying condition, this decoction is commonly used for hypertension with accompanying symptoms of headache, insomnia and a reddened tongue with yellowish fur. These symptoms, by TCM diagnostic methods (see Chapter 6), are consistent with the presence of endogenous wind with internal heat.

Summary of qi, phlegm and wind

We note that all three concepts of TCM — *qi*, phlegm and wind — represent abstractions of physiological phenomena in human bodies, albeit abstractions of different orders. The principal comparisons are summarised in Table 4.2.

---

[105] Tang (2003:277).

Table 4.2   Comparisons of *Qi*, Phlegm and Wind.

	Qi	Phlegm	Wind
Form	Formless	Sometimes liquid/solid as in sputum, but possibly formless in the stomach and organs	Formless
Substance	When stored in organs	Sputum is a substance, but other forms of phlegm are ambiguous	Never a substance
Energy	Exists at times as vital energy	Never in energy form	Appears to have energy to move like *qi*
Flow	Must flow to function	Obstructs *qi* when stagnant	Flows to cause harm

It would appear that the concepts of *qi*, phlegm and wind were invented and modified over time with Chinese medical theory to take on the roles needed to explain the functioning of the body and the illnesses caused by deviations from the body's healthy balanced state and its restoration by particular kinds of herbal agents.

Qi evolved to be a catch-all concept for all normal functioning of the body that involves change and movement. To account for the body's ability to produce *qi* continuously, the idea of storage in substance form in the organs was also necessary; hence *qi* is also portrayed in some contexts as a substance.

The concept of phlegm was associated with symptoms that were persistent (sticky like sputum) and the tendency to cause obstructions (of *qi*, blood and body fluids); certain herbs seemed to be able to alleviate these symptoms and were classified as phlegm-resolving herbs. As many illnesses are persistent and were understood to be the result of obstructions (for example obstruction of *qi* flow in the spleen and stomach, causing dyspepsia), phlegm came to be associated with many illnesses, *ergo* the conclusion that phlegm causes a hundred ailments.

Wind, on the other hand, is the pathogen that causes harm by movement. Hence illnesses with sudden onset, with dizziness and convulsions, tend to be attributed to wind.

From a biomedical standpoint, there is no reason to believe that any of these pathogens exists in a specific form that could be isolated and allow its properties to be properly recorded (other than sputum as a coagulated form of phlegm). In this narrow sense, they are convenient fictions of scientific anti-realism. Yet each is consistently associated with clearly defined symptoms that in principle have biomedical correlates. In fact, one of the interesting areas of research in Chinese medical universities today is the search for biomedical markers that define a specific TCM condition, like the presence of phlegm, a deficiency of *qi* or the movement of wind.

4.6 Conclusion

My interpretation of the ontological status of TCM entities has some similarity to that of the noted writer of Chinese medical apologetics Ted Kaptchuk at Harvard Medical School. Kaptchuk's classic *The Web that has no Weaver: Understanding Chinese Medicine* insightfully points out that the tendency of Chinese thought is to "seek out dynamic functional activity rather than to look for the fixed somatic structures that perform the activities."[106] I would add that Chinese thought is less concerned with ontology than with functionality. Whether there is an underlying real entity called *qi* with many physiological manifestations, or *qi* is merely a convenient theoretical construct for interpreting physiological phenomena does not matter to the practitioner of TCM, even if it is interesting to the philosopher. The important medical

---

[106] Kaptchuk (2000:76).

question is whether, once thus interpreted, predictions can be made and clinically tested.

Kaptchuk also likens Chinese medical theory to poetry, not to be understood literally:

> In the West, since the scientific revolution, a theory must rest on a provable physical substratum of repeatable events and measurable facts. Each fact holds up the next level. William Harvey helped usher in this scientific revolution when [...]. he overthrew the classic Greek notion of blood movement [...]. The entire Greek medical edifice crumbled [...]. Hard and substantial facts were to be the basis of the new knowledge. Qualities had to be reduced to quantities [...] speculation to experimentation. The Chinese theories, however, resemble those of Greek antiquity. This type of fact is speculative interpretation. For the Chinese, it is a sensory image, a poetic exploration of what is going on. The value of the Chinese theories is in aiding the organisation of observation, discerning patterns, capturing interconnectedness and qualities of being. Can one prove a poetic image? It can be shared. It can be used.[107]

I agree that TCM entities are interpretations, but am not sure that they are speculative or poetic, although admittedly from a pedagogical point of view this may be a good way for a new reader to be initiated into TCM entities without having to struggle with the conflict between the literal descriptions of these entities and the reader's understanding of modern anatomy and physiology. I shall argue in Chapter 6 that TCM theory, as crude and as largely unproven by the standards of contemporary evidence-based medicine as it may be, is structured as heuristic empirical scientific models that are in principle testable. TCM entities are theoretical constructs that enable the formulation of

---

[107] Kaptchuk (2000:97–98).

TCM theoretical models. TCM entities represent a different way of organising them for use in heuristic models. A similar view may be taken of anatomical systems in the body comprising vital organs and the meridians.

The entities in the TCM picture of the human body portrayed in medical texts are abstractions of anatomical and physiological realities. They look like the convenient fictions of the scientific instrumentalist, but are better understood as constructs of reality to employ in empirical models. Although terms like blood and phlegm are used to denote entities that resemble their referents in modern medicine, in fact they are part of an attempt to incorporate all the essential functions of the body within a simple framework built on a small number of entities. By ascribing diverse functions to these basic entities, TCM is able to employ them in relatively simple models for the diagnosis and treatment of illnesses.

The relevant question is whether this system of healing works well enough to be useful, and for what kind of ailments. That is the subject of Chapters 6 and 7.

Chapter 5

Organ and Meridian Systems

The kidney is the pre-natal foundation of life, and the spleen
the post-natal foundation of life.

Ancient Chinese text

According to the TCM picture of the human body, there are two core systems — the vital organs and a complex network of meridians (*jingluo* 经络). I present below a way of interpreting that theory in the light of modern knowledge of anatomy and physiology. While the description here of the TCM theory of organ and meridian systems is brief, more depth and analysis is provided for certain organs for purposes of illustrating the kind of arguments adduced with regard to their ontological status and their biomedical correlates.

The term 'meridian' is used here rather than 'channels and collaterals' only because it is shorter and more convenient. Translators who prefer 'channels and collaterals' to 'meridians' object to the latter because it could mislead the reader into thinking that they have fixed regular paths like the great circles covering the globe. In the light of the diversity of ways of translating TCM terms that I discussed in Chapter 2, this objection may not be of much practical relevance, and I have chosen the use of meridians for its terminological convenience.

As pointed out earlier, organs in TCM are different from organs with the same names in modern anatomy. To emphasise this distinction and in the interest of clarity, one could put quotation marks around the TCM organ name (e.g. 'spleen'), or italicise it (*spleen*) to indicate that it is a TCM organ. However, as nearly all references in this book are to TCM organs, it would be less tedious to leave them without italics or quotation marks. However, when I refer to the organ in the modern anatomy of Western medicine, I shall flag this to the reader with an appropriate qualification.

TCM organs are divided into two categories, the five *zang* 脏 organs (e.g. the liver) that store *qi* and other entities, and the six *fu* 腑 organs (e.g. the small intestine) that are hollow and process food and body fluids as these pass through them. The ontological status of organs has some ambiguity in TCM literature. At the time that the *Neijing* was written, little was understood about human anatomy as we now know it. Because of the prohibition of dissections of the human body in China, physicians tended to focus their attention on the external manifestations of organs through their presumed physiological functions. The result was that functions were ascribed to a number of key organs in such a way that they fitted an overarching model of human physiology and pathology (which would include the Five Elements Model, to be described in Chapter 6.) For example, the kidney in TCM theory is involved not only in excretion but also in such diverse functions as growth, ageing, warming the body, sex drive and reproduction.

Typically, TCM textbooks would refer to organs sometimes as somatic structures and at other times as 'functional units'. One textbook begins by describing the organs as somatic structures: "the five *zang*-organs and the six *fu*-organs are different from each other in functions and characteristics," but later clarifies that the concept of *zang-fu*-organs in TCM is "quite beyond the range of anatomical morphology" as the functions of the *zang-fu*-organs not only include part of the functions of organs with the same names in modern medicine but also cover certain functions of other related organs: "Obviously the *zang-fu*-organs in TCM are not just conceptions of anatomy but synthetic functional units." [108]

By "synthetic functional units" the author seems to be trying to say that TCM models of human physiology have ascribed functions to these organs that are at variance with modern knowledge of these organs. Such ambiguous treatments of organs is symptomatic of the tension between old concepts based on the *Neijing* of organs as somatic structures with multiple physiological functions and modern anatomy and physiology which have established quite different sets of functions for the somatic structures bearing the same names.

I first describe below the organs and meridians as they are presented in standard TCM texts used to train TCM physicians, then follow these descriptions with interpretations of their meanings in modern biomedical terms and of their epistemic credentials.

5.1 TCM Organs

In accordance with the Chinese medical classification, the body's organs are divided into five solid storage organs known as *zang* (脏) and six hollow organs known as *fu* (腑) paired up as shown in Table 5.1.

---

[108]Wu (2002:42, 44).

Table 5.1   *Zang-Fu* Pairing.

Zang	Fu
Liver (*gan* 肝)	Gall bladder (*dan* 胆)
Heart (*xin* 心)	Small intestine (*xiaochang* 小肠)
Spleen (*pi* 脾)	Stomach (*wei* 胃)
Lung (*fei* 肺)	Large intestine (*dachang* 大肠)
Kidney (*shen* 肾)	Bladder (*pangguang* 膀胱)

A sixth *fu*-organ called *sanjiao* 三焦 or the 'triple energiser' is essentially the trunk of the body from thorax to abdomen.[109] It does not pair with any of the *zang*-organs, but for symmetry, TCM theory incorporated the *xinbao* 心包 or the pericardium as a quasi-organ in the *zang* category. The pericardium is conceived of as a tissue surrounding the heart to protect it from pathogenic factors. In modern anatomy, the pericardium is the outer membrane that encloses the heart to which the major blood vessels emerging from the heart are attached. The significance of the pericardium in TCM will become apparent later when we discuss the 12 meridians, as each meridian is deemed connected to one of these vital organs.

The *zang*- and *fu*-organs are paired in the sense that they act in concert and support one another. For example, the spleen (*pi*) and stomach (*wei*) are both involved in digestion, and are usually jointly referred to by the compound noun *piwei* 脾胃. Likewise, the kidney and bladder act together in excretion, one processing and the other storing urine before it is passed out from the body.

The functions of the *zang*-organs are described below together with a brief mention, where appropriate, of the role of the

---

[109] It is called the 'triple energiser' because it is divided into three parts, the upper, middle and lower *sanjiao*, forming a continuous conduit for the flow of *qi* and energy.

matching *fu*-organ. Two *zang*-organs, the spleen and the kidney, are examined in greater detail to illustrate how I interpret organs and their functions within TCM theory.

5.1.1 *The spleen* (*pi*)

The spleen in TCM theory is totally unlike the spleen in modern anatomy. It is described as being "located in the abdomen" and "govern[ing] transportation and transformation" (*yunhua* 运化) as well as "command[ing] blood" (*tongxue* 统血).[110] It is the source of *qi*, blood and body fluid and thereby 'the post-natal foundation of life' (*houtian zhi ben* 后天之本). In this respect, its role contrasts with and is complementary to that of the kidney, which stores *qi* and *jing* ('essence') inherited from parents and is therefore regarded as the pre-natal foundation of life' (*xiantian zhi ben* 先天之本). (*Jing* will be described further below.)

The stomach works in concert with the spleen in digestion. The function of the stomach in TCM is "to receive and digest food; the chyme[111] transformed in the stomach is then transmitted to the small intestine".[112] This is quite similar to the stomach in modern anatomy whose function is to continue the process of digestion that begins in the mouth; its digestive juices and churning action reduces the food to a semi-liquid partly digested mass that passes on to the duodenum.[113]

The TCM description of the spleen's function as governing transportation and transformation calls for further explanation. We first consider the meaning of 'transportation and transformation';

---

[110] Wu (2002:62–63).
[111] 'Chyme' is the "semi-fluid mass of partly digested food expelled from the stomach into the duodenum" (*Webster Collegiate Dictionary*).
[112] Wu (2002:75).
[113] Oxford (2007:682).

the significance of 'govern' in Chinese medicine will be separately discussed further below in Section 5.2.

5.1.1.1 *'Transportation and transformation'*

In essence, this means transforming food and water into nutrients that are then transported to the organs and muscles of the body. The standard TCM textbook description of how this takes place appears somewhat complicated and ambiguous. One text begins by saying that "the spleen can digest food, absorb nutrients of food and water, and then transport them to the heart and the lung," but goes on to say that "food is digested and absorbed by the stomach and small intestine but it must depend on the transporting and transforming function of the spleen to transform [it] into nutrients which, relying on the functions of the spleen to transmit and disperse essence, are distributed to the four limbs and other parts of the body".[114] The tendency for TCM texts to incorporate modern knowledge of physiology into TCM theory can lead to inconsistencies, for example saying that "food is digested by the stomach and small intestine" while maintaining the Chinese classical description that the spleen governs transformation and transportation of food, nutrients and water.

The problem could lie in the classical portrayal of the role of the spleen in digestion, spelt out in terms that border on the metaphysical: 'the spleen *governs* (*zhu* 主) transportation and transformation', as if it were some kind of sovereign entity that orchestrated and regulated the digestive work done by the stomach, small intestine and other organs of the body. The mechanism by which the spleen governs is laid out in detail by classical

---

[114]Wu (2002:62).

texts as well as modern texts and revolves around *qi*. The transforming and transporting function is divided into two parts: transporting and transforming food nutrients, and transporting and transforming water. Food that is absorbed though the stomach and small intestine must depend on the spleen-*qi* to transform it into an intermediate substance called 'nutrient essence' (*jingwei* 精微) which is dispersed to the four limbs and other parts of the body. The rest of the water absorbed from the food nutrients is transported by the propelling function of spleen-*qi* to the lung and kidney where it is transformed into sweat and urine to be excreted out of the body. If spleen-*qi* is sufficient for the transporting and transforming functions to be executed, the organs receive enough nutrients and exhibit vitality; when spleen-*qi* does not perform its functions adequately, the body is an unhealthy state and symptoms of abdominal distension and pain with loose stools may appear; dampness and phlegm retention can occur, with the accompanying symptoms of dizziness and lassitude.

In addition to governing transportation and transformation, the TCM spleen also 'commands' blood by confining it to the blood vessels and preventing it from flowing to outside tissues. This aspect of the spleen is at variance with modern physiology for which the spleen is a major component of the recticuloendothelial system, producing lymphocytes in the newborn and containing phagocytes that remove worn-out red blood cells and other foreign bodies from the bloodstream. It also acts a reservoir for blood.[115] In ordinary language, the spleen in modern physiology helps clean blood and stores it, quite different from being the governor of digestion and the commander of blood.

---

[115] Oxford (2007:673).

5.1.2 *Interpreting the functions and ontological status of the spleen*

The legendary physician Li Dongyuan of the Song dynasty paid great attention to the spleen in health cultivation and therapy, basing much of his medical skills on the management of spleen functions. His classic *Treatise on the Spleen and Stomach* has been a reference manual for generations of Chinese physicians even up to the present day. This manual focuses on the spleen's transforming and transporting functions by which it replenishes primordial qi (*yuan-qi*) in the kidney, thus making the spleen the fountain of post-natal health. If the functions of the spleen are compromised through illness, excessive emotion and/or poor living habits, the body undergoes progressive deterioration as each organ begins to fail from lack of nourishment.

What is the biomedical equivalent of the spleen? As pointed out earlier, and also alluded to in the literature on Chinese medical anthropology,[116] ancient Chinese thought often not only fails to distinguish clearly between somatic structures and functions; it also tends to blur the distinction between substance and energy (as in conceptions of *qi*), between entities and processes (for example, the five elements are also known as the five phases) and between attributes and substances (*yin* and *yang* are attributes as well formless substances).

Viewed in this light, the spleen in TCM is a set of functions closely related to the biomedical concepts of digestion and absorption of food and water and the distribution of nutrients and liquids to the organs and tissues of the body. By identifying a somatic structural organ to incorporate these functions, TCM theory has clustered them in such a manner as to fit with TCM

---

[116] See, for example, Farquhar (1994), Kleinman (1995) and Julien (1995).

models used for explaining observable physiological phenomena and for the diagnosis and treatment of illnesses. From the point of the evolution of Chinese medical thought, it is likely that the ancients thought, incorrectly as we now know, that the somatic spleen had all these functions, as even a casual reading of *Neijing* would lead one to conclude.

As knowledge of anatomy and physiology advanced, particularly in the post-1949 Chinese revolution when Chairman Mao instructed the modernisation of Chinese medicine by drawing on the knowledge of Western medicine, it would have become apparent that the functions associated by ancient Chinese medicine with the various organs were inaccurate, if not grossly wrong. A shift to the idea of the organ as a representation of a set of functions would have been the only escape, short of giving up most of TCM theory, given that so much of the theory of diagnosis and therapy had already been built upon these functions.

Pragmatically, it does not matter for the practice of Chinese medicine that these functions are clustered together under the same names as the somatic structures of modern anatomy, or even that we imagine these structures really had these functions. The key to understanding the cluster of functions ascribed to a particular organ is that, as a theoretical construct, it must fit into models of health, diagnosis and therapy in Chinese medicine. *The TCM organ is thus the result of organising functional activities and classifying them in such a way as to be consistent with and usable in TCM models.*

In the case of the spleen and stomach, between them these organs have to capture the processes of digesting and absorbing food and distributing nutrients to the rest of the body.

In addition, herbal tonics for a weakened spleen (manifested by digestive problems) were found to be useful for treating conditions such as hematuria (blood in the urine), hematochezia (blood in the stool), uterine bleeding and subcutaneous purpura, thought to be attributable to a reduced ability for blood to be confined to the blood vessels. The role of the spleen in 'commanding blood' would be consistent with these empirical observations.

Thus the spleen is, in effect, not an organ with functions, but the functions themselves. This may be the best way to interpret the awkward term "synthetic functional units" that we came across earlier in the TCM textbook explanation of organs. In sum, the spleen is a theoretical construct that captures various aspects of digestion and distribution of nutrients and water described in modern physiology, as well as the function of keeping blood within blood vessels.

As the functional activities of the spleen are driven by spleen-*qi*, the use of herbs and acupuncture techniques in promoting health and in treating illness naturally make reference to their beneficial effects on spleen-*qi* (as well as the related stomach-*qi*). The action of herbs and acupuncture in relation to the spleen can broadly be divided into (a) being a tonic to strengthen spleen-*qi*, commonly abbreviated to "*tonifying* spleen-*qi*" [117]; (b) assisting in the flow of *qi* (*regulating qi*). The main difference between (a) and (b) is that one is concerned with the stock of stored *qi* and the other with its smooth and unimpeded flow. To use an automotive analogy, tonifying *qi* fills up the tank whilst regulating *qi* clears blockages in the fuel line and carburettor.

A deficiency in spleen-*qi* can compromise the spleen's functions of absorbing and transforming food, leading to inadequate supply of nutrients to the rest the body and manifesting in lassitude, a bloated abdomen and loose stools. When there is poor regulation of *qi*, water retention tends to develop, leading to symptoms associated with internal dampness and phlegm. One

---

[117] The word 'tonify', uncommon in English usage, is used extensively in the translated TCM literature to denote 'using a tonic for'. I have followed this practice throughout the book.

way to interpret these disorders of the abdomen is that weakened spleen-*qi* or impediments to its flow are responsible for poor digestion, abdominal discomfort and many of the symptoms associated with the irritable bowel syndrome. TCM theory has taken such a pattern of abdominal disorder and attributed it to the malfunction of spleen-*qi*.

As we shall see in the next chapter, this is expressed in TCM models as patterns of illness (syndromes) being differentiated and ascribed to a malfunctioning spleen-*qi* mechanism. The ontological status and physical properties of spleen-*qi* is not an issue in TCM theory, but therapeutic models based on these interpretations of the spleen are claims that should be testable if they are to be regarded as scientific.

As with the earlier interpretations of the nature of TCM entities, spleen-*qi* is in effect defined by certain patterns of symptoms when it is deficient or its flow is impeded, just as the spleen itself is defined by the functions it is presumed to have. Any biomedical investigation to isolate spleen-*qi* and determine its physical properties, in the way one might isolate a body secretion and examine its cellular and chemical composition, is inappropriate. Likewise, a biomedical interpretation of the spleen as being the combination of a number of organs like the stomach, small intestine and the pancreas, all of which are known in modern physiology to be involved in digestion, is also inappropriate as it would stem from the erroneous notion of spleen as a somatic structure or a combination of several such structures.

Different categories of herbs and acupuncture procedures are used for tonifying and regulating (promoting the flow of) *qi*. Qi tonics are among the most common in Chinese pharmacopeia. Among the general *qi* tonics are ginseng and Astragalus, whilst tonics specifically useable for spleen-*qi* are *dangshen* (*radix codonopsis*), *baizhu* (*rhizome atracylodis macrocephalae*) and *gancao* (liquorice).

For the regulation of spleen-*qi*, *jupi* (dried tangerine peel), and *xiangfu* (*rhizome cyperi*) are often prescribed.

Which came first in TCM theory? The spleen as an organ with specific functions or the observation that certain herbs have the ability to resolve symptoms of illness like poor appetite, lassitude, abdominal distension and loose stools that the theory associates with a dysfunctional spleen? The *Neijing*, with detailed and extensive passages on functions of the spleen and other organs, preceded Zhang Zhongjing's *Treatise on Febrile Diseases*, the first medical manual to list a wide array of important herbal prescriptions that today form the foundation for formulations used by Chinese physicians. This might suggest that the functions of the spleen were established first and the herbs for treating the spleen identified later. More likely, however, they evolved together. The *Neijing* was written and rewritten by more than one person during the 400-year history of the Han dynasty. A great deal of clinical practice would have preceded any written codification and clinical observations of the outcomes of different herbal treatments must have helped shape the theory.

It is evident from case studies of physicians and ancient texts that TCM theory evolved gradually over time through clinical experience and experimentation with herbs and formulations. There were no dramatic breakthroughs like Koch's culture of the *tubercle bacillus*, Pasteur's development of vaccines, Fleming's discovery of penicillin, or Watson and Crick's double helix model of DNA structure. Arguably the only conceptual breakthrough happened two thousand years ago when Chinese medical thought abandoned the idea of spirits and numinous agents as the cause of illnesses and the casting out of spirits as the cure for them. The *Neijing* laid down the empirical basis for Chinese medical science by tracing causal factors of illness to the outside natural environment and the body's host environment, especially the prevalence of harmful emotions. Models that led to diagnostic techniques and therapeutic methods based on herbs and/or acupuncture were then developed.

TCM uses the same approach to understanding and interpreting the functions of the kidney and the other organs.

5.1.3 *The kidney (shen)*

Besides excretion, the kidney (*shen*) in TCM plays a central role in growth and reproduction; it is also regarded as the source of stored *qi*, *jing*, body warmth, marrow and brain matter, and to house the ability to resist illness. So wide and varied are the functions of the kidney that many pathological conditions are attributable to a disorder of some aspect of kidney functions.

In effect, the kidney is the seat of youth and vitality. This explains why so much of the TCM approach to preserving good health in middle and old age has to do with protecting and boosting the functions of the kidney.

The main physiological functions of the kidney to be found in TCM texts are stated briefly below, followed by an explanation of their intended meanings within TCM theory and, finally, an interpretation of the theory. The functions are:

1. Governance of growth and development;
2. Governance of reproduction;
3. Governance of water;
4. Governance of *qi* reception *qi*;
5. Production of marrow to enrich the brain and transform blood;
6. Nourishment and warming of the viscera.[118]

---

[118]Wu (2002:65–70).

In explaining how the kidney carries out these functions, TCM theory makes extensive use of the concept of essence or *jing*, thought to be a substance stored in the kidney. Yet, the nature of *jing* is hard to define or understand. It is usually given only brief mention in introductory TCM texts although it is dealt with at length in the *Neijing*.

Jing in TCM is the key substance involved in development. One inherits a fixed amount of it from parents and draws it down through life. This is termed *pre-natal jing*. *Post-natal jing*, on the other hand, is produced from the synthesis of food and environmental forces, and the cultivation of emotional wellbeing and the intellect. An interesting Western interpretation of *jing* captures well this idea in beautiful poetic terms: "Essence is the quality or texture that imbues an organism with the possibility of development, from conception to death. Essence is also responsible for the development of the deepest awareness and wisdom."[119]

I take the more secular view that *jing* represents ancient Chinese thought's struggle with the notion of a person's genetic make-up (nature) and the effect of post-natal influences (nurture) on his physical and mental development.

Interestingly, post-natal *jing* in Chinese medicine has a corollary meaning: semen, usually treated as an external visible manifestation (materialisation) of kidney-*jing*, just as sticky phlegm coughed out from the lungs is a visible materialisation of phlegm. As semen, *jing* is greatly emphasised in Taoist manuals of health that advocate its conservation (in sexual intercourse through withholding ejaculation) to enhance vitality and longevity.

The kidney also stores *qi*, *yin* and *yang*; these substances are similarly regarded to be involved in growth and development. If

---

[119] Kaptchuk (2000:57).

the kidney has a deficiency of *qi,* or a deficiency/excess of *yin* or *yang,* development may be affected.

The reproductive function of the kidney is related to growth and development. *Jing, qi, yin* and *yang* of the kidney are involved in growth, the onset of puberty, menstruation, and maintaining differences between the physiology of men and women.

The kidney governs water in the sense of controlling the amount of liquid in the body by participating in its transportation within the body and in excretion through the bladder. 'Water' is used in the sense of pure water; if it contains waste substances it is 'turbid'. TCM describes the filtering action of the kidney as '*qi*-transformation' by which it separates out the 'lucid' part of the water and 'elevates' it to the heart and lungs, while the rest is transformed into urine and transported to the bladder.

The kidney's function in the 'reception of *qi*' (*naqi* 纳气) refers to its receiving (processing) of fresh *qi* from the air inhaled by the lung and storing it. It also participates in respiration in the sense that it acts in concert with the lungs to ensure that respiration results in the various organs and tissues receiving enough air (*qi*) for them to carry out their work. TCM classics as well as modern texts use the term '*gushe*' 固摄 (fixate) for the role of kidney-*qi* in receiving *qi* from the lung, and guiding its transport to the kidney, bringing about respiration. The lung is thus said to 'govern respiration' but it can do so properly only with the cooperation of the kidney. If kidney-*qi* is weak in the body, disorders like shortness of breath and asthma are thought to be possible outcomes.

Kidney essence (*jing*) produces marrow (*sui* 髓) which, in TCM, has a wider meaning than it has in modern physiology. It includes bone marrow, the spinal cord and 'cerebral marrow' in the brain. Marrow nourishes the bones, while the spinal cord together with brain marrow nourishes the brain. The brain is recognised in TCM as a separate organ that governs the five *zang*-organs, mental activities and the motion of the limbs. If there is deficiency of kidney essence, cerebral marrow production is impaired and pathological changes such as headache, dizziness, amnesia and retarded response to external stimuli may result.

Kidney essence is also thought to be transformable into blood and therefore constitutes a source of blood in addition to that derived from the digestion and transformation of nutrients by the spleen. Blood can also be transformed into (post-natal) kidney essence.

Finally, the kidney in TCM nourishes and warms the viscera (i.e. the *zang*- and *fu*-organs). Kidney-*yin*, also known as primordial *yin* (*yuanyin* 元阴), nourishes the *yin* of all the viscera and also supplies them with *yin*-fluid. The concepts of viscera *yin* and *yin*-fluid are peculiar to TCM, capturing the idea that organs need to be nourished and bathed in fluids to keep them functioning strongly. Kidney-*yang*, also known as primordial *yang* (*yuanyang* 元阳), warms the viscera. *Yin* and *yang* in the kidney have to be in balance for the body to be in good health. Deficiency in one leads to a corresponding deficiency in the other *zang*-organs. For example, a deficiency in kidney-*yin* leads to deficiency of liver-*yin*, heart-*yin* and lung-*yin*, and a deficiency in kidney-*yang* brings about deficiency of spleen-*yang* and heart-*yang*. On the other hand, deficiencies of *yin* and *yang* in other viscera can also deplete the kidney of its own stock of *yin* and *yang* and, if sustained and prolonged, leads to the "exhaustion of the kidney" and the eventual impairment of all five *zang*-organs.[120]

It can seen from the above that the kidney in the TCM theory of health cultivation plays a central role in the promotion and maintenance of vitality and hence in fostering longevity. One

---

[120]Wu (2002:70–71).

can thus understand why Chinese tonics have largely revolved around the kidney for growth, sexual activity, reproduction, resistance to cold weather, and delay of the ageing process. Together with the spleen, it forms the foundations of life. This is the basis for the aphorism that the kidney and spleen are respectively the pre-natal and post-natal foundations of life.

5.1.4 *Interpreting the kidney in TCM*

As in the case of the spleen, the kidney as an 'organ' in TCM is really a cluster of functions, indeed a veritable hodgepodge of apparently unrelated functions.

Why the ancients thought it fit to make the kidney the repository of so many functions is an interesting question, but mainly for the Chinese medical anthropologist. It may have something to do with the kidney of Western anatomy, situated towards the back of the body around the waist area, being the site of soreness following vigorous sexual activity, and with a chronic aching back being a leading indicator of physical decline that comes with ageing, *ergo* the sexual, reproductive and growth functions of the kidney.

Alternatively, as I observed in the discussion of the concepts of wind and phlegm in the last chapter, the clustering of processes sometimes has to do with the herbal medications that have been found to work on a family of apparently unrelated conditions; the conclusion is thereby drawn that these conditions arose from the same origin. Kidney-*yang* tonics like cordyceps, deer horn (*pilose antler*) and *shenqiwan* pills (肾气丸) are recorded in the Chinese pharmacopeia as sex tonics, but are also used for the prevention of premature greying as well as the treatment of children who are slow in growth and development. This clustering of uses, which might appear to have no theoretical basis from the standpoint of biomedicine, could have arisen in TCM simply from clinical practice in which the same medications appeared to be effective for these different uses, hence the functions that were being treated with the medications were grouped together under the kidney.

What biomedical science now terms the genetic characteristics of an individual were in effect held by Chinese theory to be carried in pre-natal essence (*jing*). The storage of *jing* in the kidney and its role in growth and reproduction would appear then to quite naturally fall into place.

The connection between the kidney and the brain is a little harder to explain. One conjecture would be that Chinese medicine observed that the neurological aspects of motion, thinking and sensory perception are controlled by the brain, and these functions decline with age. As the TCM kidney governs ageing as a phase of growth and development, it would make sense to cluster brain functions with kidney functions.

Finally, we note that the urinary function of the kidney in TCM seems to have little to do with the other kidney functions in the cluster. Why then did Chinese medicine put them together? My conjecture is that the Chinese discovered the sexual functions of the adrenal glands covering the superior surface of the kidney. To the unobservant eye of those in China involved in illegal dissections, the gland could have been regarded as part of the kidney. The cortex of the adrenal gland is derived embryologically from the mesoderm (the middle germ layer of the early embryo) and is stimulated by the pituitary gland (which regulates post-natal growth) to produce various hormones, among which are those secreted by the sex glands, mainly oestrogen and androgen. An association between the kidney and sex and reproduction would therefore be quite natural. A more imaginative explanation would be that for men urine is discharged through the same orifices involved in sex and reproduction, and in adjacent orifices for women.

For the sake of completeness, I shall deal with the other three *zang*-organs albeit somewhat cursorily as the descriptions of the TCM understanding of the spleen and kidney are already sufficiently rich for the purpose of illustrating how TCM organs differ so radically from organs in modern anatomy yet providing a plausible basis for a biomedical interpretation of TCM organs. I have made only passing mention of the *fu*-organs as these tend to be closely associated with their corresponding *zang*-organs and discussion of the *fu*-organs and interpreting their functions would not add to the basic approach of understanding the ontological status of organs in TCM.

5.1.5 *The liver (gan)*

The principal activity of the liver in TCM is to 'dredge and regulate' (疏泄), which is the idea of clearing and smoothing the routes along which *qi* flows, as well as regulating the flow and activity of *qi*. It is a concept peculiar to TCM. In Chinese therapy, *shugan* 疏肝, meaning 'dredging and regulating the liver' is used for problems in liver function. 'Soothing the liver' is the more common alternative translation for *shugan*.

By regulating the activity of *qi*, the liver also regulates the activities of all other vital organs and tissues. Among the implications of this principal function of the liver is that it promotes circulation of blood and metabolism in the body, and it also assists the spleen and stomach in digestion. As with the liver in Western medical anatomy, the liver also stores blood.

5.1.6 *The heart (xin)*

The heart in TCM has two main functions: to 'govern blood' and to control the mind. The first function is similar to the function of the heart in Western medical physiology, in the sense that it propels blood to circulate in the vessels; but it also has the implication that the heart is involved in the production of blood. The second function implies that the heart stores an entity called 'spirit' (*shen* 神), which has the function of cognition and consciousness. In this sense, the functions of the heart in TCM include the mental functions of the brain in Western medical physiology.

5.1.7 *The lung (fei)*

The lung has the function of governing *qi* by controlling respiratory movement as well as regulating *qi* activities in the body. This includes the production of pectoral-*qi* (*zong-qi*). The lung in TCM also regulates water passages in the body for transmitting and discharging water, thereby propelling, adjusting and excreting water from the body. Another important aspect of the lung is that it assists the heart in blood circulation. In TCM theory, blood from vessels converge in the lung and is redistributed to the rest of the body; hence the *Neijing*'s famous aphorism: 'The lung is connected to all blood vessels' (*fei chao baimai* 肺朝百脉). This has implications for the Chinese interpretation of lung cancer as it is consistent with a malignant tumour in the lung tending to metastasise more readily than other tumours and to spread to the bones, brain and liver.

Chinese medicine views the body as an organic whole, hence the functions of organs do not exist in isolation but must always be understood in relation to other organs and the network of meridians that connect them. The principal model that connects the organs is the Five Elements Model (to be covered in the next chapter).

5.2 On 'Governing' (主)

The preceding paragraphs have put forward the case for treating an 'organ' in TCM as a cluster of functions. Historically these functions were ascribed to a physical organ recognisable in modern anatomy as a somatic structure. Modern TCM texts tend to be ambivalent, sometimes referring to the organ in modern anatomy while at other times treating it as a 'synthetic functional unit', thereby shifting emphasis to functions. There is a possible tension between classical Chinese thought, which believed that the physical organs had these functions, and modern TCM theory, which can scarcely ignore the biomedical evidence for the proven physiological functions of these organs. Such tension is totally unnecessary once we interpret the TCM organ as an abstraction that represents a cluster of functions or, more simply, treat an organ as the cluster of functions.

This tension is reflected also in the ubiquitous reference in Chinese medical literature to an organ as 'governing' a number of functions. The word 'govern' is the translation of '*zhu*' 主 which in Chinese has several meanings. As a noun, *zhu* 主 can denote the guest–host relationship as in *binzhu* 宾主 ; it can refer to the master–servant relationship as *zhupu* 主仆 it is also the term for the monotheistic God. As a verb, *zhu* can mean 'manage' as in *zhuguan* 主管 (manage an organisation); it can mean 'advocate' (a cause), or 'propose' (a course of action). In modern TCM texts, *zhu* is translated into English as 'govern', implying that the somatic structure acts like a master directing certain activities in the body. Thus when TCM says that the kidney governs growth and development, the implication is that this organ directs its stock of *jing*, *qi*, *yin* and *yang* to carry out tasks in accordance with the biological program built into its pre-natal essence. Using the notion of governing like a human-like person directing operations in the body helps conceptualise physiological activities.

Such use of language is similar to the use of the term 'design' in describing functionality in biological teleology. One approach to functionality in evolutionary biology is to separate the notions of design and function as in:

1. X is a biological function of T and
2. T is the result of a process of change of structure due to natural selection that has resulted in T being better adapted for X than ancestral versions of T.

For example, to say that an eagle's wings are *designed* for soaring is to claim that the ability to soar explains why some ancestral eagles had higher reproductive fitness than others, and that eagles' wings are better adapted for soaring than were those of their evolutionary ancestors.[121]

Design can also imply the existence of a human designer, or a spiritual one if we subscribe to religious teleology. In biomedical science, the designer is the adaptive process of evolution among living organisms, orchestrated by the principle of natural selection. The designer is the natural selector.

Similarly, when we say that the spleen governs transformation and transportation, we give human-like status to an organ which in fact is no more than an abstraction of the physiological forces that combine in some orderly manner to bring about absorption and digestion of food and water and their transportation to other parts of the body. How the functions came to be clustered in this particular manner is a matter of historical interest. In most instances it was influenced by lack of anatomical

---

[121] Borrowed and adapted from the Stanford Encyclopedia of Philosophy.

understanding, such as the combination of the kidney and adrenal glands as one organ. In all likelihood, the clustering was also influenced by cosmological models from which ancient Chinese models drew inspiration. For example, the number of key *zang*-organs was limited to just five to fit the Five Elements Model, and organs like the brain, pancreas and uterus had to be relegated to a special class of 'extraordinary organs'.

Orthodox thinkers in Chinese medicine hold the ancients in high regard as they are deemed to have gained divine insight into the workings of the body through cultivated introspection.[122] That they hold such beliefs does not necessarily imply that their diagnosis and prescribed therapy for a patient would be different from that of a modern TCM practitioner who pragmatically follows the same models because he thinks that they work for his purpose and does not particularly care about how those models came about.

The pertinent question is whether or not such a system of clustering serves a useful medical purpose: Does it yield diagnoses that can be used to administer effective therapies? Chinese medical practitioners have found that such a clustering of functions when applied with TCM models seems to be usable for their clinical work. Of course, whether in fact these models do indeed work should be and can be subjected to clinical trials.

Failure to understand the meaning of organs and their functions is the cause of considerable confusion among those who adhere to the literal interpretation of Chinese medical entities and systems and see this as in conflict with the findings of biomedical science, resulting in unnecessary internal tension in their thought processes. TCM physicians who have not learnt to resolve this conflict need to make what one observer terms "epistemological leaps" as they try to mediate ancient wisdom and

---

[122] Liu (2003:14–16).

biomedical knowledge in their daily practice.[123] The arguments I have presented here offer a way out of this conflict.

5.3 Meridians and Collaterals

The 'meridian system' (*jingluo* 经络) in TCM theory is a network of passages that transports *qi*, blood, *jing*, *yin* and *yang* throughout the body.[124] It connects the *zang*-organs among themselves and with their counterpart *fu*-organs, and links all other parts of the body including the bone, skin, muscles and tendons and the nine orifices, allowing the body to function as an organic whole.[125] The system also maintains communication between the body and its external environment by carrying information signals as well as energy and materials derived from nature, thereby achieving a balance between the body and its host environment. The meridian system is therefore much more than a neurological network that enables the acupuncturist to treat pain by inserting needles into appropriate points in the network. So broad is the concept of the meridian system that the functions sometimes claimed for the system rival those of the organ system in importance.

The term 'meridian' is used in two ways in TCM theory. It could refer to the entire system, or it could refer to the main trunk routes in the system; the context of use usually makes it clear which is being referred to. The meridian system (*jingluo* 经络) comprises main trunk routes, the meridians (*jing* 经)

---

[123]Lo (2002:Introduction, xlix).

[124]It is not entirely clear in what ways the blood that flows in the meridians is different from blood that flows in blood vessels. Chinese thought seems not to have differentiated between the two but regard them as playing complementary roles.

[125]The nine orifices comprise the eyes, nose, ears, mouth, and the sex organ and the anus.

and smaller branches called collaterals (*luo* 络) that criss-cross to form an intricate network. The meridians run at the level of muscles and organs and hence at a deeper level than the collaterals, which mostly run at the level of or just below the skin. All the meridians, with the exception of the *dai* (带) meridian, run vertically, and the *dai* meridian runs transversely around the body.

The meridians in TCM are analogous to roads and highways that link villages, cities, farms, and industrial installations in a country. They have an existence in their own right: they contain *qi* and can become diseased when invaded by pathogens, or they can develop obstructions that hinder the flow of *qi* and communication signals along them. The meridians therefore behave as if they were a parallel set of organs; they can become ill or dysfunctional, and specific meridian-based pathological conditions can be identified.

The principal components of the network are the 12 main meridians (*jingmai* 经脉) and eight 'extraordinary' meridians, commonly translated as the eight 'extraordinary vessels' (*qijing bamai* 奇经八脉). Each of the 12 main meridians is connected to a particular organ and is named after that organ. Hence one speaks of the spleen meridian, the bladder meridian, and the like. The five ordinary *zang*-organs together with the pericardium make up six *zang*-organs matching six *fu*-organs, each of which would be connected to one of the 12 main meridians. The six meridians associated with the *zang*-organs are deemed to be *yang* in nature, and the others associated with the *fu*-organs *yin* in nature. These classifications reflect the Chinese propensity for balance and symmetry. Among other things, the *yang* meridians run along those parts of the body that face the sun (the back and the outside of the limbs), while the *yin* meridians are on the chest and the inside of the limbs, which are usually shaded from the sun. The meridian associated with the *sanjiao* (triple energiser) *fu*-organ is paired with the pericardium meridian.

The eight 'extraordinary vessels' have no direct connection to the *zang* and *fu*-organs. The most commonly used extraordinary vessels for therapy, particularly acupuncture therapy, are the governor vessel (*dumai* 督脉), the conception vessel (*renmai* 任脉), and the thoroughfare vessel (*chongmai* 冲脉). The *dumai* is thought to 'govern' the *yang* meridians and the *renmai* the *yin* meridians. The *chongmai* is termed 'the sea of blood' as it is deemed to be the place where all *qi* and blood in the body converge.

The relevance of the meridians in TCM goes far beyond therapy for pain. Their main use lies in their association with and connection to particular organs. For example, acupuncture needles applied to points along the spleen and stomach channels can have a tonifying effect on these organs, hence they are often used for patients with digestive disorders. Acupuncture of points along the *renmai* and *chongmai* are used to treat gynaecological problems as there is thought to be a connection of these extraordinary vessels to the uterus.

Despite their importance within the TCM theoretical framework, in practice, the meridian functions are not emphasised as much in diagnosis and therapy as are those of the organ system. This may well be because there is enough in the TCM framework involving the organs and the basic entities of *qi*, blood and body fluids to cover most cases of diagnosis and treatment. Emphasis on the use of meridian theory to diagnose and treat disease probably reached its height shortly after the publication of Zhang Zhongjing's *Shanghan Lun* (*Treatise on Febrile Diseases*) in the Han dynasty. Today many of the febrile conditions identified by the *Shanghan Lun* are named after the associated meridians, such as *taiyang bing* (太阳病), a condition arising from injury to the small intestine meridian, but their diagnoses and treatments use herbs that address the concomitant *qi* and organ disorders.

5.4 An Interpretation of Meridians

Among practitioners of acupuncture, a distinction is made between TCM acupuncture and *Western acupuncture.* The latter is used somewhat loosely to refer to acupuncture carried out by those who follow the scientific method established by Galileo and others in the 17th century when they introduced "systematic verification through planned experiments to the existing ancient methods of reasoning and deduction".[126] The basic idea of Western acupuncture is that the diagnosis should follow the principles of Western medicine: treatment efficacy should be verified through clinical trials, and physiological accounts should be found for the mechanism by which needling imparts therapeutic effects. As I shall argue in the next two chapters, given an appropriate interpretation, TCM theory in general and acupuncture in particular are not at odds with science. Its major methods and practices can in principle be the subject of clinical trials, albeit not always in accordance with the requirements of a generation of medical scientists brought up on the ideology of randomised controlled trials being the only acceptable protocol for evidence-based medicine.

Using evidence-based methods, much work has been done on the physiological interpretations of Western acupuncture and on identification of points that can be used for specific therapies. The result has so far been that many of the acupuncture points (acupoints) identified by TCM acupuncture coincide with

---

[126] Filshie and Cummings (1999:31).

myofascial "trigger points"[127] but Western acupuncture does not generally subscribe to the configuration, indeed to the existence, of the meridians used in TCM.[128] Conjectures regarding the efficacy of needling are made in neurophysiological terms, for which there is a burgeoning literature triggered by President Nixon's visit to China in 1972 when television documentaries of surgical operations conducted on fully conscious patients treated with acupuncture needles.[129]

For pain relief or acupuncture analgesia, biomedical explanations have focused on neurophysiological and neuropharmacological mechanisms.[130] The discovery of transferable analgesia from animals treated with acupuncture to untreated animals by cross-circulation of blood and cerebrospinal fluid led to more intensive research into a cast of neurophysiological players like endorphins, serotonin and encephalins.[131] Placebo effects are thought to be equally powerful and are the subject of extensive research.[132]

In sum, Western acupuncture has offered biomedical explanations for its alleged efficacy, and it has been extensively subjected to clinical trials. It does not depend on the TCM theory of meridians. In contrast, meridians play a central role in TCM acupuncture as

---

[127] The term 'myo' is a descriptive for muscle; 'fascia' pertains to the fibrous membrane separating muscles and also forming the layer between the skin and the muscles. See Taber's Cyclopedic Medical Dictionary (2001:775).

[128] Filshie and Cummings (1999:38–42).

[129] See for example Ernst and White (1999). These procedures have since been challenged and there have been claims that other analgesia/anaesthesia may have been involved. What is not in doubt is that they captured the attention of the medical world and aroused an interest in acupuncture.

[130] Various explanations of the mechanism of acupuncture are offered separately in papers by Lundeberg, Birch and Hsieh in Hong (2013).

[131] See Filshie and Cummings in Ernst and White (1999:36).

[132] See, for example, Hong (2013), Kaptchuk (2000) and Evans (2003).

needles are usually inserted into selected acupoints that lie along one or more of the meridians.

Historically there has been sustained Western interest in the nature of meridians — whether they exist and, if they do, whether they are neurological networks, paths of low resistance to flows of energy, or the paths for some other kinds of flow. The meridians, conceived as a physical network like nerves and blood vessels, have never been isolated, nor has their biomedical nature been determined despite many attempts by Chinese and Western scientists. Lu and Needham reported in 1980 that attempts to demonstrate a physical or sub-anatomical substratum for the system were inconclusive.[133] Leung *et al.* cite other hypotheses in 2003, including one postulating them as low electrical impedance paths, none of which have been confirmed.[134]

Within TCM theory, there are two distinct questions over meridians that are of interest. The first concerns its role to convey *qi* and blood and its use to relieve pain. Pain in TCM theory has to do with obstructed flow, as captured in the aphorism 'where there is no flow there is pain; when there is no pain, there is flow' (*butong ze tong, butong ze tong* 不通則痛, 不痛則通). The TCM explanation is that the acupuncture needle stimulates the flow of *qi* and blood. Pain is therefore mitigated by promoting better flow with a needle at the locus of pain or, more commonly, at a receiving point and transmission point along one of the meridians.

The second aspect of meridians is their connection to the organs and their therapeutic use for illnesses associated with the organs. For example, TCM theory would prescribe acupuncture on points along the spleen and stomach meridians to stimulate the production and flow of spleen-*qi* and stomach-*qi*, which are

---

[133] Lu and Needham (1980:186).
[134] Leung *et al.* (2003:176–177).

needed to alleviate problems of digestion, bloated stomach, or lack of appetite. This function of the meridians is the more important one for TCM theory as it is an integral part of the overall holistic framework of explanation for illness, diagnosis and therapy.

In the light of the TCM concept of the organs as a set of functions rather than somatic structures with fixed loci, the notion of meridians physically tracing their paths to the site of organs becomes suspect, and the conventional maps showing the intricate paths of each meridian with an endpoint in a (Western anatomy) organ could conceivably come to grief. An escape from this dilemma is to interpret the meridian maps as being merely schematic once a meridian enters the visceral region, where it somehow interacts with the functions of the organ with which it is supposedly linked. This is not entirely satisfactory and a consideration of the ontological status of meridians seems appropriate.

My conjecture is that the intricate network mapped out in ancient Chinese texts, which continues to be used by modern TCM physicians in clinical work, does not exist as a set of physically isolatable pathways. Attempts to map the network using electrochemical and other techniques are likely to be doomed to failure, for the same reason that it does not make sense to isolate *qi*, phlegm and wind for chemical analysis. The meridian system is an explanatory model that experience has found to be useful in the sense that in clinical situations the body behaves *as if* these pathways existed when the physician applies his needle. The biochemical mechanisms, as has been found from recent research on pain treatment with acupuncture, are vastly complex and unlikely to be adequately captured in a system of 12 meridians and eight extraordinary vessels. [135]

---

[135] See "The Ontological Status of Meridians" in Hong (2013).

As some Western researchers speculate, the ancients found that pressure on certain points led to pain relief in other areas of the body and, based on their belief in the flow of *qi*, proceeded to map out paths to explain those effects.[136] Over time, these putative paths grew into a large network, parts of which may have been merely hypothesised and not subjected to testing in clinical work. The result was an unwieldy meridian network. One should add that in one of the *Neijing*'s volumes called *Lingshu*, many organ disorders were treated with pressure with fingers or sharp stone implements on acupoints, and a holistic picture emerged which reflected the influence of Chinese cosmological models. These emphasised symmetry and correspondence; in particular, the Five Elements Model led to the association of meridians with the *zang*-organs.

The truth of the matter in clinical practice is that experienced acupuncturists constantly improvise new acupuncture points that may not be related to the mapped meridians. These are known as '*a shi*' (阿是 or 'Oh yes!') acupoints, based on the experienced acupuncturists eliciting positive responses from their patients when their needle hits a sweet spot. These *a shi* points would appear to have little relation to the meridian system.

To ancient medical thinkers, the human body was a black box whose content could only be conjectured on the basis of its external manifestations. Models of the workings of the internal component systems in the black box were invented by observing output responses to inputs. These models were often guided by Chinese cosmology and a rich metaphysical poetic tradition, as well as the belief that the human body was a microcosm of the external universe. This is a subject of the next chapter.

---

[136] Filshie and Cummings (1999):32.

Chapter 6

TCM Models in Explanation and Prediction

It does not matter if a cat is white or black as long as it catches mice.

Deng Xiaoping

A modern interpretation of Chinese medicine must aim to (a) show how TCM theory may be reconstructed to be understandable from the vantage point of biomedical science and (b) assess the evidential credentials of the thus reconstructed theory.

Toward the first aim, I have argued that TCM entities are a combination of real entities and theoretical/fictional constructs, and that the systems of organs and meridians are merely ways of classifying and organising physiological activities to fit into the models of TCM theory. This reconstruction of TCM theory departs from the classical interpretation of all TCM entities as real and organs as somatic structures as in modern anatomy.

In this chapter, I present the key models of TCM theory, not as immutable laws of nature, but as *heuristic* models found from clinical experience to be useful guides for diagnosis and therapy. I examine a number of key models in TCM theory and interpret them wherever possible from a biomedical standpoint, thereby taking the second essential step towards reconstructing TCM theory. In the next chapter, I address the second aim of the book, showing how and to what extent TCM evidential credentials may be evaluated through clinical trials and case studies.

Before examining the principal models used in TCM it is necessary to consider the concepts of *yin* and *yang* that lie at the base of much of Chinese philosophy and Chinese medical theory.

6.1 *Yin-Yang:* The Principle of Balance as the Basis for Health

The concepts of *yin* and *yang* were introduced in distant antiquity, before Taoism and the *I-Ching* or *The Book of Changes* (circa 600 BC). There are extensive discussions of *yin* and *yang* in the *I-Ching* and it undoubtedly was a major source of philosophical insight in Taoism, which gave it full expression in poetry, metaphysics, statecraft and medicine.

The ideas of *yin* and *yang* in Chinese philosophy and medicine are usually presented as *Yin-Yang Xueshuo* (阴阳学说), the doctrine (or theory) of *yin* and *yang*. The doctrine reflects a dialectical logic that attempts to explain relationships and change. Stripped to its bare essentials, *yin* and *yang* are not much more than labels that describe the perception of duality in nature — light versus darkness, hardness versus softness, male versus female. Thus the *yin-yang* doctrine is a way of holistic viewing of the cosmic world, a way of thinking that places all entities as part of a cosmic whole — entities that cannot have existence independent of their relationship to other entities.

Chinese medicine took these concepts from cosmology and, viewing the body as a microcosm of the universe in which ideally things are in harmony and balance, it regarded human health as being based on a balance between *yin* and *yang* in the body. As such, the *yin-yang* doctrine is not so much a scientific theory as it is a conceptual framework for the models in TCM theory. The models themselves are used for explanation and prediction and, if they claim to be scientific models, must be capable of yielding testable hypotheses.

The basic idea of *yin* and *yang* is simple and might appear to be an unlikely source of medical wisdom. Dualism of natural states and attributes means that an attribute like brightness has meaning only relative to darkness, as does beauty relative to ugliness.[137] Objects and states can be similarly classified: day and night, summer and winter, hard and soft. Attributes come in contrasting pairs: male and female, transparency and murkiness, and so on as the sample in Table 6.1 illustrates.

The correlation of these attributes to male and female stereotypes is rather obvious. Social stereotypes can be similarly viewed. For example, Nisbett classifies the West with its predilection for

Table 6.1   *Yin* and *Yang* Attributes.

Yang	Yin
Strong	Mellow
Bright	Dim
Rigid, unyielding	Flexible, yielding
Hard	Soft
Transparent	Unfathomable
Hot, dry	Cool, moist
Fast, hurried	Slow, patient
Analytical	Discursive
Insensitive	Sensitive

---

[137] Laotze, the founder of Taoism, explains it in terms of recognition of attributes: "It is because everyone under Heaven recognises beauty as beauty that the idea of ugliness exists." (*Daodejing*, Chapter 2, line 1)

transparency and the rule of law as *yang* and the East with its penchant for subtlety and flexibility as *yin*.[138]

Yin and *yang* are attributes but also substances in the human body; for example, we speak of the *yin* and *yang* as substances in the kidney, but also of *jing* (essence) as a substance with *yin* attributes, and *qi*, a substance with *yang* attributes: each is deemed stored in various organs. This blurring of distinction between substances and attributes, and also between action and physical state, is common in ancient Chinese thought and often reflected in the grammar of the Chinese language. For example, the word *gandong* 感动 can be a verb, meaning to move someone emotionally, or a noun to denote the action of moving someone, or an adjective describing the person's emotional state of being moved. *Yin* and *yang* are attributes in some contexts, but in other contexts they are substances having *yin* and *yang* characteristics. This apparent disregard for ontology needs to be borne in mind when evaluating Chinese medical theory, which is influenced by the emphasis of ancient Chinese thought on functions and processes rather than on the physical nature of the underlying entities.

While a balance of *yin* and *yang* is the ideal in nature, there have been philosophical debates over which was intrinsically stronger (much as the West has had debates over which is the weaker sex among human beings). Legend has it that the debate over which was mightier, *yin* or *yang*, was settled by Laotze when the young moral philosopher Confucius made a long journey to have an audience with the older sage in the latter's declining years to seek guidance on the subject. Laotze had little time for Confucian moral absolutism, believing instead in going with the flow and a balance of all extremes. He was a man of few words, the extant record of his entire philosophical output being a tract

---

[138]Nisbett (2003).

of a mere 5,000 words, the *Daode Jing*. When Confucius raised the *yin-yang* question, the aged sage cast him a disdainful look, opened his mouth wide and pointed his finger at his decaying oral cavity. The conversation ended there, leaving Confucius profoundly puzzled. Only the long track back to his lodgings cleared his mind: Laotze's hard teeth were all long gone but the soft tongue was alive and well.

The Chinese regard for *yin* carries over to medical thought: gradual cures are more lasting than quick fixes; soft methods will eventually triumph over hard ones; the nourishing of *yin* is, in most instances, a better way to go than tonification for *yang*, and the soft graceful movements of *Taiji* shadow boxing in misty country air superior to vigorous aerobic exercises in a bright urban gym.

Certain principles govern the relationship between *yin* and *yang*. They complement each other but also oppose each other, a combination of mutual support and check and balance. The idea of mutual dependence and mutual opposition is captured in the classic graphic presentation of *yin* and *yang* (Fig. 6.1). *Yin* and *yang* wrap around each other, providing mutual support but each also holding the other in check.

Yin is needed for generation of *yang* and vice versa. For example, blood (a *yin* substance) is needed for the production of *qi*

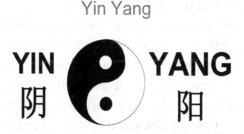

Fig. 6.1 Graphic Presentation of *Yin* and *Yang*.

(a *yang* substance), and *qi* is also involved in the production of blood. *Qi* is also the driving force for the movement of blood.

Yin and *yang* wax and wane. For example, in the diurnal cycle of the world outside the body, *yang* starts growing stronger after midnight and by dawn it dominates over *yin*, continuing to grow until it reaches a peak at noon, then declines and gives way to *yin* which gains ascendancy after dark and peaks at midnight. A similar cycle is thought to exist in the human body, with the body rising in vigour from dawn and turning passive after dark. The seasons likewise see *yang* growing rapidly in early spring and reaching a peak in mid-summer; by the autumn *yin* is ascendant and finally reaches a maximum in winter.

The healthy body is conceived by TCM as one that is in perfect balance. Balance implies that *yin* and *yang* as mutually opposing forces are in harmonious coalition and in equilibrium. A principal cause of illness is an imbalance between *yin* and *yang*, and therapy consists in restoring balance. There have been attempts to relate the concept of balancing *yin* and *yang* to underlying biomedical processes. One of these is homeostasis, a process by which the internal environment of the body comprising such factors as temperature, blood pressure and acid-base balance is maintained in dynamic equilibrium under conditions of a varying external environment. This is achieved by an ever-changing process of feedback and regulation in response to external or internal changes.

Yin and *yang* have also been compared to *anabolic* and *catabolic* forces in body metabolism as understood in Western medicine. Anabolism is the synthesis of complex molecules such as proteins and fats from simpler ones, and an anabolic force is one that promotes tissue growth by increasing the metabolic processes involved in protein synthesis. Catabolism is the chemical decomposition of complex substances in the body to form simpler ones, accompanied by the release of energy. The substances being broken down include nutrients in food such as carbohydrates and proteins as well as storage products such as glycogen.[139] Anabolism is thought to be *yin* and catabolism to be *yang*. One claim is that every cell and every bodily system alternates between *yin* anabolic activity and *yang* catabolic activity: if a cell is excessive in its catabolic *yang* activity, then an anabolic *yin* activity will be instituted to balance the action to ensure continued healthy cellular activity.[140]

Duality in body systems such as the sympathetic nervous system (which is involved in fight/flight) and the parasympathetic system (which calms down the body) have also been compared to *yang* and *yin* forces respectively.[141]

While such comparisons may have some superficial appeal, there is little to support them beyond their being helpful analogies for TCM pedagogical purposes. Within Chinese medicine, *yin* and *yang* have clinical meaning mainly with respect to models in TCM theory that attempt to define physiological and pathological states of the body. A set of symptoms may be identified as belonging to a particular imbalance. For example, 'weakness of kidney-*yang*' is a condition that arises from *yang* being weaker than *yin* in the kidney functional system, possibly the result of poor nutrition, overwork or sexual excess. It manifests itself in symptoms of lassitude, a pale complexion, fear of wind and cold, a thin pulse, chronic back pain, frequent urination and sexual dysfunction. The treatment is with *yang* tonics for the kidney. (The role of *yin* and *yang* in clinical diagnosis and in the choice of therapies will be clearer when we deal with *differentiation of syndromes* further below.)

---

[139] *Oxford Concise Medical Dictionary* (2007).
[140] http://www.drmarkholmes.com/pdf/Homeostasis.pdf, retrieved 12.23.2013.
[141] http://drlwilson.com/Articles/CATABOLISM.HTM, retrieved 12.23.2013.

The *yin-yang* principle does not amount to very much more than the common observation of dualism in nature, that attributes mostly come in pairs. The mutual dependence of *yin* and *yang* for generating each other can be seen as the need for some kind of homeostasis-like equilibrium in physiological functions. As for the waxing and waning of *yin* and *yang*, these were originally derived from the cyclical character of natural phenomena — the diurnal cycle, the seasons and circadian rhythms of the body. They became useful tools for analysis of the workings of the body, and their meanings expanded as early medical thinkers tried to explain physiological phenomena inside the body. TCM models use these concepts to capture what were perceived to be attributes of various entities in the body and their dynamic states.

6.2 Principal TCM Models

The term 'model' as used in science, and in the philosophy of science, has many meanings, and is sometimes a source of confusion. In this book, I use this term only because it facilitates reference to observed or postulated regularities in TCM theory. Chinese medical classics hardly if ever use this term. However some modern interpreters of TCM theory have used the concept of the model to characterise the theory's basic principles and observed regularities. Zhang Qicheng, for example, regards TCM theory as 'model-based quasi-science' (*moxing kexue* 模型科学) and eschews the classical view of TCM theory as comprising inviolable natural laws into which ancient wisdom had somehow gained special insights.[142]

There is no universally accepted definition of a model. Frigg and Hartmann describe models as one of the principal instruments

---

[142] Zhang (1996, 1999).

of modern science, lament the "incredible proliferation of model-types in the philosophical literature", but stop short of defining the term.[143] Psillos calls it a "term of art used in understanding how theories represent the world."[144] Duhem, Mach and others held that theoretical models in science are merely dispensable aids to theory construction and can be "detached and discarded" when the theory is fully developed whilst Campbell sees models as analogies that are essential parts of theories, as in the case of the theory of gases which uses the model of point particles moving like billiard balls at random in the vessel containing the gas.[145] Such analogies might merely serve as inadequate stepping stones to better theories, as was the case when statistical mechanics eventually learnt to stand on its own two feet and the billiard ball model was no longer needed.

In the social sciences, particularly in economic science, models are used to represent idealised situations that approximate to real economic conditions at particular places and times. For example, Adam Smith's model of economic efficiency in competitive markets holds true provided that the conditions for perfect competition exist. These include free markets, absence of state intervention, perfect information, and the absence of transaction costs. In the demand-supply model, consumers are pictured as seeking a fictitious entity called "utility", yielding an equation for an objective function to be optimised under supply and budgetary constraints.

For the purpose of reconstructing TCM theory, which can be viewed as having a number of models associated with it, it is convenient to use that term in a similar manner to Ronald Giere. A scientific theory comprises a cluster of models, together with a number of hypotheses about real things claimed to be similar to

---

[143] Frigg and Hartmann (2006).
[144] Psillos (2007).
[145] Hesse (1967:357).

one or another of the models. "A theoretical hypothesis is [...] a statement asserting some sort of relationship between a model and a designated real system [...]. Hypotheses, then, claim a similarity between models and real systems."[146]

Whether TCM models qualify to be called *scientific* models must then depend on whether hypotheses regarding illnesses can be derived from these models and whether these are testable in principle, preferably also in practice. To establish the scientific nature of TCM models, one must therefore be able to present testable hypotheses based on these models. This must mean that the methods of diagnosis and treatment can be put to clinical test. If these hypotheses can be put to the test, the claim that TCM is scientific can begin to be made. Testing may well lead to a rejection of much of TCM theory. However if some parts of the theory were confirmed through hypothesis testing, it would give TCM more scientific credibility although, like economics and evolutionary biology, it would probably never enjoy the same level of acceptance as theories in the physical sciences because of its complexity and the practical (but not insurmountable) difficulties of conducting clinical trials.

Giere's allowance for similarity rather than a strict correspondence between models and what they represent coheres with my view that TCM theory comprises mainly (crude) heuristic models that, like many models in the economic and the social sciences, are thought to be useful for practical purposes, even though they do not seem to work *all* the time. (Witness the successes and failures of Keynesian economics in different times and economic environments.)[147]

---

[146] Giere (1988:80).

[147] However, I do not necessarily subscribe to Giere's more radical position that science can do without laws of nature, arguing that "it is models, not laws in the traditional sense, that do the important representational work in science". Acceptance of this viewpoint is not essential to adopting his framework of theories, models and hypotheses. See Gierre (1999) *Science Without Laws*.

It is worthwhile reiterating at this point that in describing TCM theory as using models that may be put to scientific test, one should not regard TCM itself as a science or a potential science. Like architecture, engineering and economic management, TCM is a *practice* that makes use of the knowledge that science offers. It is a human enterprise to heal disease and promote health. It makes use of (alleged) science, employing what it believes to be scientific models just as the profession of architecture uses physics and chemistry to design structures and select building materials. Unlike the physical and biological sciences, TCM does not primarily seek the truth and reality underlying natural phenomena. Instead it tries to find rules and regularities in nature that help explain health and illness and employs suitable methods to achieve its objective to heal illness and promote human health. In this respect, it is not different from modern Western medicine.

A cluster of models together collectively make up the theory of TCM. Some key models are examined below.

6.2.1 *The five elements: The model of physiological interaction*

Wuxing (五行) is translated as 'the five elements' or 'the five phases' depending on whether one takes it to describe relationships among substances or relationships among dynamic processes. For example, one of the main applications of the model is in relation to the five *zang*-organs, which in TCM usually represent clusters of functions but are sometimes treated like somatic structures. I shall use the term 'five elements' as it is more common in the translated literature.

Wuxing Xueshuo (五行学说) is usually translated as the *theory* of the five elements. However, '*xueshuo*' more commonly means 'teachings', implying that there may be a doctrinal aspect to it.

Hence it is also translated as the Doctrine of the Five Elements. I call it the *model* of the five elements, in line with my view of TCM theory as comprising heuristic models.

The Five-Element Model is related to ancient thinking that all things in the natural world are derived from the basic elements of wood, fire, earth, metal and water. The model places wood, fire, earth, metal and water consecutively in a clockwise ring combination to capture their mutual relationships and interactions. Each *zang*-organ is associated with one element, and elements and organs are matched up as follows: wood-liver, fire-heart, earth-spleen, lung-metal and kidney-water. The model thus places the five *zang*-organs in the same ring combination (Fig. 6.2).

The model describes relationships among the five elements that can be applied to the selection of therapeutic methods in TCM. The first relationship is that of 'promotion' (*sheng* 生). Each organ promotes the one next to it in the clockwise direction in the sense of nourishing, strengthening, or 'giving birth to' to it, and in that sense it is the 'mother' of that organ. For example, 'earth promotes metal' implies that strengthening the spleen is one way of nourishing and tonifying the lung. A patient with weakness in his lung (functions) can be treated with a spleen tonic, which in turn strengthens the lung to overcome imbalances within that organ. In TCM clinical practice, this is indeed

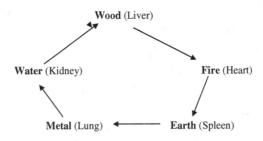

Fig. 6.2   The Five Elements Model.

one of the most commonly used therapies for lung problems. By nourishing the spleen (digestive system), a weak lung can be strengthened. This approach is especially useful for patients who, for one reason or another, are unable to accept medication directly for lung disorders: giving tonic to the spleen would more gently build up their lung functions. There is a similarity here to Western practice, in the pre-antibiotic age, for which diet was the major component in the regimen for treating consumption (tuberculosis of the lung).

The second main relationship in the five-element model is that of 'restraint' (*ke* 克). Each element restrains the next one two steps down the clockwise ring; for example, wood (liver) restrains earth (spleen), and fire (heart) restrains metal; in familial terms, grandmother restrains the grandchild. In the healthy human body, this acts like check and balance: mother promotes the child, whilst grandmother guards against excesses in the grandchild. This relationship is useful in TCM for explaining instances when restraint is overdone. For example, an excess syndrome ('exuberance') of the liver, which may be induced by pent-up anger or excessive consumption of alcohol, suppresses (over-restrains) the functions of the spleen, causing it to underperform its functions. It also suggests that certain problems of the spleen arising from over-suppression by the liver can be treated by 'calming' the liver.

The five-element model has long been a pillar of Chinese medical thought, but in recent decades it has become the subject of debate. It has been estimated that in reality about half of the permutations of relationships among the organs implied by the five-element theory are not used in clinical practice, probably because they have not been found to work.[148] For example, a method of tonifying a weak spleen termed 'strengthen fire to

---

[148] See Ou (2005)

tonify the earth' (*yihuobutu fa* 益火补土法) would, by the five-element model, imply strengthening the mother heart organ to tonify the spleen. In practice, this is rarely done. Another source of 'fire' is deemed to be the kidney which also has a warming function for the rest of the organs. In clinical practice, physicians strengthen kidney *yang*, rather than the heart, to tonify the spleen; this is not in accordance with the five-element model.[149]

Another example of inconsistency within the five-element model is the common method of 'mutual reinforcement of metal and water' (*jinshui xiangsheng fa* 金水相生法) for treating deficiency in lung-*yin*, a condition common in dry autumn weather in Northern China and occurring in post-influenza dry coughs generally. Besides directly nourishing lung-*yin*, the five-element model would prescribe that the physician should also strengthen the mother organ of the lung (the spleen). Instead a 'mutual reinforcement of metal and water' unrelated to the five-element model prescribes strengthening kidney-*yin*. The rationale behind this is that the kidney is believed to be a source of *yin* for all organs.

Such inconsistencies have led prominent Chinese medical thinker Deng Tietao at the Guangzhou University of Chinese Medicine to advocate that the five-element model be modified to the more practical "the five-organ set of relationships", which merely sets out those relationships among organs that are thought to be useful based on clinical experience without the constraint of conforming to some ancient cosmological model.[150] This in effect amounts to giving up the five-element model and instead just setting out a list of those relationships among the

---

[149] It is instead in accordance with the *mingmen* or 'gate of life" theory which places the kidney in the central role of warming the body's organs. See Wu (1995) *Zhongyi jichu xue*, 31.

[150] Deng (1988).

organs that have been found to be helpful in clinical practice. Such a step would replace an ancient model drawn from cosmology with a more practical one based on empirical experience. This change would support my view of TCM models as heuristic models derived from empirical findings rather than principles based on ancient cosmological laws.

6.2.2 Climate and emotions: The model for illness causation

Ancient Chinese texts cite six exogenous (climatic) factors and seven emotions as causes of disease (or pathogenic factors). Modern TCM texts add toxic chemicals, microbiological agents (viruses, bacteria, fungi, etc.), parasites and harmful dietary and living habits. Although it recognises the existence of microbiological agents, modern TCM practice defers to Western medicine to deal with these matters and views climatic and emotional factors and poor dietary and living habits as providing the *grounds* for the invasion of these agents to cause illness. As noted earlier in Chapter 2, this understanding of causation is in accord with the Chinese medical emphasis on the value of prevention over cure. Hence, protection against adverse climatic influences and moderation of one's emotions are the key principles for the cultivation of health; from a biomedical standpoint they may help prevent harmful microbiological agents from affecting the body.

Climatic influences are usually referred to as the six exogenous factors (六淫): Wind (风), cold (寒), summer heat (暑), dampness (湿), dryness (燥) and fire (火).

When these climatic factors invade the body and are not expelled, they can become internal pathogenic factors with characteristics similar to their external counterparts. We have also dealt with their endogenous counterparts bearing the same names (in Chapter 3).

Wind is blamed for the largest variety of illness. It is characterised by movement; hence a form of rheumatism with pain moving to different parts of the body is thought to be due to wind within the body. Cold and heat in the weather have parallels internally in pathological conditions of heat and cold. Summer heat is extreme heat (fire) often accompanied by dampness as well. Dampness is high humidity when it is external and is associated with symptoms of stickiness (being difficult to eliminate) when it penetrates the superficies, slowing a person down and causing stagnation in digestion when it is present in the spleen. Dryness, on the other hand, is present typically in the autumn and winter months in temperate countries and air-conditioned rooms in the tropics.

The seven emotions (七情) in TCM are pleasure, anger, anxiety, grief, fear, shock and melancholy, of which the first five are more commonly encountered. Each of the seven is thought to be associated with a specific *zang*-organ (see Table 6.2).

'Pleasure' here refers to excessive indulgence in pleasurable activities, including excessive sex.

Table 6.2   Emotion-Organ Association.

Emotion	Organ(s) damaged by this emotion
Pleasure	Heart
Anger	Liver
Anxiety	Spleen
Grief	Lung
Fear	Kidney
Shock	Heart
Melancholy	Lung, liver

Anger damages the liver, which explains why a sudden fit of anger can cause wind or fire to rise from the liver to the head and cause headaches, dizziness, red eyes or elevated blood pressure. Likewise, frequent anger stirs up the liver, manifested in 'wind' that travels to the head (possibly causing hypertension and strokes) or suppression of the spleen, causing gastric disorders.

'Anxiety' is often translated inappropriately as 'contemplation' but is more correctly interpreted as constant and unremitting thinking and worrying (brooding), a state which I prefer to call (chronic) anxiety. It acts slowly on the spleen, gnawing away at one's health at the basic level of digestion and nutrition. It is the most insidious and damaging form of emotion, wearing down the body and eventually leading to more serious illnesses as the other organs are affected by the poor functioning of the spleen. The incidence of disorders of the spleen tends to be higher in societies and in professions where there is pressure for achievement and people are constantly and often unconsciously in a state of anxiety. (They look at their smart phones at meal times and allow them to intrude freely into time spent with friends and family.) This is manifested in such problems as the irritable bowel syndrome, bloated stomachs and general dyspepsia.

Grief damages the lung and TCM explains that this is the reason we sigh a lot when stricken with grief.

Fear affects the kidneys and is thought to be the reason that extreme fear can cause incontinence and also affect the reproductive function and damage fertility.

In practice, the climatic-emotional model for causation of illness is useful more as a guide to cultivating health rather than for diagnosis or treatment. As we shall see below, diagnosis and treatment revolve around recognition of patterns of symptoms that are manifested by the underlying disorder.

6.2.3 *Syndromes: The model for diagnosis and therapy*

The 'syndromes' model for diagnosis and therapy is central to TCM theory and constitutes an important distinction between biomedicine and TCM. The former emphasises the diagnosis of diseases and etiology (usually specified at the level of blood components, cells, genes and micro-organisms) whilst the latter is focused on discerning constellations of symptoms that are classified into patterns of illness known as 'syndromes' or *zheng* (证). *Zheng* is also translated as 'pattern' or 'manifestation'. We shall use 'syndrome' as the more common translation.[151]

The TCM syndrome or *zheng* (证) has similarities to, but is fundamentally different from, a syndrome in Western medicine. The latter is "a combination of signs and/or symptoms that forms a distinct clinical picture indicative of a particular disorder": for example, the chronic fatigue and irritable bowel syndromes.[152] As will be explained further below, a TCM syndrome is one of a number of defined recognisable patterns. It is not a disease in the Western medical nosological sense. It may be associated with more than one disease, and a disease can exhibit different syndromes in the course of its progression (pathogenesis), hence the aphorism 'different treatments for the same disease, same treatment for different diseases' (*tongbing yizhi, yibing tongzhi* (同病异治，异病同治).[153] For example the syndrome of *qi* weakness is a common condition in coronary heart disease, but may also be observed in patients with stomach ulcers. A disease can be

---

[151] See Farquhar (1994), Scheid (2002:201) and Sivin (1987:109).

[152] *Oxford Concise Medical Dictionary* (2007): A syndrome is "a combination of signs and/or symptoms that forms a distinct clinical picture indicative of a particular disorder", e.g. chronic fatigue syndrome.

[153] The translation of 'disease' here for *bing* (病) is not totally satisfactory as the Chinese *bing* has a wider meaning that includes the universe of disease *and* illness in the Western sense as described in Chapter 2.5).

associated with different syndromes, and these syndromes can change over time as the disease progresses. For example, tuberculosis is a disease with symptoms of blood in the sputum, daily fevers, lassitude, and loss of weight. A person with the disease might exhibit *yang* deficiency in the lung at one stage and *qi* stagnation of the spleen at another. These require different TCM treatment regimens, even if the patient was concurrently being treated with the same Western antibiotics throughout these stages.[154]

The identification of syndromes in a patient through a process of diagnosis recognising the patterns associated with the syndrome(s) is termed *bianzheng* 辨证 (differentiation of syndromes). The therapy administered is termed *lunzhi* 论治 (applying principles of therapy). Combining the two, the model of diagnosis and treatment, central to TCM theory, is *bianzhenglunzhi* 辨证论治, or 'differentiation of syndromes and treatment accordingly'.

There are several classification systems for the differentiation of syndromes, but the commonly used ones are:

(a) *bagang* 八纲: classification by the eight principles or the eight basic syndromes
(b) *zangfu* 脏腑: classification by the visceral system

---

[154] Scheid (2002:207) notes that while the differentiation of syndromes was discussed in various parts of the *Neijing* and *The Treatise on Febrile Diseases*, and were used at various times in the history of Chinese medicine, there was also emphasis on diseases and symptoms in addition to syndromes. It was only in the Republican era that, under the influence of classifications seen in biomedicine, TCM underwent the "wide-scale systematization of the presentation of diseases, patterns and symptoms and signs" that was needed to make differentiating syndromes a distinguishing feature of contemporary Chinese medicine.

(c) *wei qi ying xue* 卫气营血: classification by the level of penetration of the pathogen, at the superficies, *qi*, nutrient *qi* and blood levels

(d) *qi xue jingye* 气血津液: classification by *qi*, blood or body fluid being involved

(e) *bingyin* 病因: classification according to external climatic causes — heat, cold, dampness, wind, etc.

(f) *liujing* 六经: classification by the six meridians

Some Western writers, notably Sivin, Farquhar and Kaptchuk, prefer to use more exotic terms like "the eight rubrics", "the four sectors of the warm illness school" and "the six warps" for (a), (c) and (e) respectively.[155]

Modern textbooks usually explain that the different classification systems can be used together, mutually supplementing one another.[156] Historically, however, there have been rivalries among various schools of thought. For example, the six meridian system is emphasised by the 'Cold Damage School' (*shanghai xuepai* 伤寒学派) based on the *Treatise on Febrile Diseases,* while the 'Warm Disorders School' (*wenbing xuepai* 温病学派) favours the *wei qi ying xue* system. As Ren Yingqiu puts it, all schools of thought are derivatives of the basic tenets of the *Neijing* and have varying emphases that reflect the living environments at different historical periods and in diverse geographical regions.[157] For example, the warm pathogens school became influential in late Ming and Qing dynasties when medical thought was stimulated by studies by Wu Youxing (1582–1652) of infectious diseases common in spring and summer in the south. This became a competing school of thought to the cold damage school of the *Shanghan Lun*

---

[155] Sivin (1987), Farquhar (1994) and Kaptchuk (2000).

[156] Wang (2002:2).

[157] Ren (1986).

from the ancient Han dynasty when climate-related illnesses were brought about largely by exposure to winter cold.

In practice, several of the classification systems are used simultaneously to differentiate a syndrome. Typically, a syndrome is differentiated by specifying the locus of the illness and the state of the body at that locus. The locus could be a viscera, in accordance with (b) above, or meridians (e), or generalised throughout the body at a certain level of penetration (c) and involving a particular substance or fluid (d). The state of the body is described by one or more of the eight basic syndromes in *bagang* (eight rubrics) comprising: exterior and interior, *yin* and *yang*, heat and cold, and deficiency and excess. 'Exterior' in this instance refers to the locus of illness being at the level of the superficies, and 'interior' refers to the rest in increasing depth, from *qi* to blood.

The concepts of heat/cold and deficiency/excess are different from those of ordinary language. 'Heat' in TCM has little to do directly with temperature. It is a basic syndrome defined by a set of symptoms — a red tongue, a quickened pulse, a redder complexion possibly with redder eyes, a feeling of warmth and vexation, sore throat and preference for cold over warm drinks. An elevated body temperature may or may not be present, and is neither a necessary nor a sufficient condition for having heat in the TCM sense.

Deficiency (*xu* 虚) and excess (*shi* 实), also translated as asthenia and sthenia respectively, are described in the *Neijing* as follows:

> When pathogenic breaths [from without] are ascendant, that is *shi*;
> When a person's essentials breaths (*jing* and *qi*) are depleted, that is *xu*.[158]

---

[158] *Yellow Emperor's Canon of Medicine* (2005:ch.28) *Suwen*. 'Essential breaths' here refers to essence (*jing*) and *qi*.

The concepts of excess and deficiency have a close similarity to those of repletion and depletion respectively in ancient Greco-Roman medicine, in which the notion of repletion is associated with over-indulgence in food and drink and depletion results from stress, sexual exhaustion, or inadequate nutrition.[159] In TCM, deficiency can also be the result of pathological processes that weaken the body, as in the case of someone who suffers from a chronic debilitating illness or has just recovered from an acute infection. The excess syndrome is also observed in TCM when the body confronts an invading pathogen and has adequate *zheng-qi* (healthy *qi*) to put up a fight. This resultant struggle between pathogen and *zheng-qi* is manifested as an excess syndrome. If however *zheng-qi* is low and the body's defences are therefore weak, the body succumbs quickly to the pathogen and exhibits a deficiency syndrome. Excess is often but not always correlated with surplus *yang* and heat, and deficiency with *yin* and cold.

In the course of the progression of an illness (pathogenesis), the prevailing syndromes are in a dynamic state and can change over time, as the following example illustrates.

A patient is subjected to cold harsh weather and his body defences break down. He catches a chill that develops into a fever. He has a runny nose, a mild cough and a headache, and is averse to cold and wind; his tongue is pale with little fur, and his pulse is 'floating'. In TCM thought, these are symptoms of 'cold damage' affecting the outer layers of the body. The patient's syndrome is 'cold at the exterior (surface) level' (*biaohan zheng* 表寒证).

At this stage, if he has sufficient *zheng-qi*, the body can be assisted to resolve the condition with a warm diaphoretic medication like the *Ephedra* decoction (*Mahuang Tang*). Essentially this decoction expels the surface cold pathogen by inducing

---

[159] See, for example, Nutton (2004), "Humoral alternatives", pp. 202–215.

perspiration.[160] The patient should achieve full recovery in one to three days.

Without treatment and proper care, his condition could progress to a more serious stage where he develops a fever and sore throat, his tongue is red with thick yellowish fur, his pulse is rapid, his face is flushed and he feels warm. His cough worsens and is accompanied by thick yellowish phlegm. The pathogen is thought to have penetrated deeper into the body, and he now has the syndrome of internal heat with dampness (*shi re li zheng* 湿热里证). Medications for clearing heat and resolving dampness would need to be administered. The recovery period would be longer. After the internal heat and dampness have cleared, he feels weak and exhausted, his face is pale, his tongue is pale red with little fur, and he has a persistent dry cough. His syndrome is that of combined deficiency of lung-*qi* and of deficiency of lung-*yin* (肺气肺阴两虚). He needs a *qi* tonic to strengthen his lung functions and a *yin* tonic to nourish the lung; the former promotes air movement in and out of the lungs, and the latter encourages secretions of body fluids (*sheng jin* 生津), moisturising the dry phlegm in his lungs and enabling it to coagulate so it can be easily coughed out as white phlegm. This tonification treatment could take over a week, or several weeks if the patient is elderly or has a weak constitution.

In the above example, the syndrome of 'cold at the exterior level' invokes the classification system (a) for cold, and (c) for exterior level. The next stage of pathogenesis was 'internal heat with dampness' which draws on (c) for internal, (a) for heat and (e) for dampness. Finally, in his weakened state his syndromes are 'deficiencies of lung-*qi* and lung-*yin*', drawing on (a) for deficiency and *yin*, (b) for viscera, and (d) for *qi*.

---

[160]TCM considers perspiration as resolving both cold and warm conditions at the exterior level. If the condition is that of heat at the exterior level, a cool diaphoretic like dried chrysanthemum flowers (*juhua*) would be used.

A physician's ability to differentiate syndromes and apply appropriate treatment accordingly requires experience as sometimes several syndromes are present and complications arise from patients having different natural constitutions (such as some tending to have more heat or more dampness than others in their normal state). Detailed guidelines are provided by a system of diagnosis and therapy, which is outlined below, albeit only briefly since our primary emphasis here is on the epistemological issues in models of diagnosis and treatment.

6.2.3.1 *The four examinations*

The method of diagnosis to enable the physician to differentiate syndromes is known as the 'Four Examinations'. The basic principle of the four examinations is to make inferences about the body's internal condition based on symptoms observable by the physician and described by the patient. In ancient times, the physician did not have diagnostic tools such as X-rays, laboratory blood tests, ultrasound and MRIs that are now the common fare of Western physicians. The modern TCM physician continues in the tradition of the ancients by relying on the four examinations to enable him to draw conclusions about the patient's syndromes. The procedure of the four examinations is akin to a mapping process in which each observation fixes a coordinate on a multi-dimensional symptom map. The overall map so derived yields a pattern that enables the physician to differentiate the syndrome.

The four examinations (*wang wen wen qie* 望闻问切) consists of:

1. inspection or visual observation (wang 望)
2. listening and olfaction (wen 闻)

3. inquiry (wen 问)
4. pulse-taking and palpation (qie 切).

Inspection (visual observation)

Inspection means observing the patient's face, tongue, the colour of his skin, the glow ('spirit') in his eye, his gait and his posture. Inspection alone yields a large number of diagnostic inputs to the experienced physician who can often do a fairly accurate diagnosis based only on inspection.

The patient's face is observed in detail for such manifestations as the colour of the skin, the presence or absence of a healthy glow, the spirit in his eyes (whether full of life, dispirited, filled with anger or sadness, etc.), and the presence of unusual growths or pigmentation of the skin. The patient's gait is also observed as he enters the physician's clinic, and anything unusual in his posture and movements is noted. His whole body is also examined if the physician deems it necessary.

The examination of the tongue is an extremely important part of the visual observation. Several aspects of the tongue are noted: its size (whether thin and withered, or swollen with tooth indentations, or normal), its colour and, very significantly, the texture and the colour of the fur on the tongue. A slightly red tongue is normal but a deeper red could indicate internal heat, whilst a dark tongue with a purplish hue is often associated with poor blood circulation and blood stasis.

A person of normal health would have thin whitish fur on the tongue. Thick greasy fur indicates presence of dampness, while unusually thin fur, or no fur at all, may imply the presence of *yin* deficiency associated with asthenic internal heat. Thick yellowish fur is usually seen when there is internal heat from an excess syndrome.

Listening and olfaction

Listening and olfaction provides additional information — the voice of the patient, any unusual odour he emits, and the sound of his breathing (being clearly discernible if he is suffering from phlegm retention in his bronchioles, a sore throat, or an asthmatic condition).

The physician listens to the patient's voice to determine if it is weak or strong, smooth or hoarse, clear or slurred. His manner of breathing, whether slow or hurried, smooth or laboured, shallow or deep, and the presence of cough are all noted. The power of his voice is an indicator of the level of his pectoral *qi*.

Inquiry

Inquiry can be a fairly long process, lasting for over half an hour for a new patient. At the first visit to a physician, the patient should be asked a long list of questions concerning his past medical history, bowel movements, urination, appetite, sleep, adaptability to hot and cold environments, aversion to wind, sexual activities, eyesight and moods. The patient is also asked to describe how he feels, and the main medical complaint that led him to consult the physician.

An experienced physician can ask penetrating questions that allow him to accurately narrow down the range of conditions with which the patient might be afflicted. In a sense, the inquiry part of the four examinations is the most challenging but rewarding one as a tremendous amount of information can be extracted from this process. Some modern Western doctors, who rely heavily on laboratory diagnostic tests and spend less time understanding how the patient feels, could be missing crucial information that can help the doctor determine the patient's condition.

Pulse-taking and palpation

Finally, pulse-taking or feeling the pulse reveals further information about the inner condition of his body. TCM differentiates between dozens of different pulses, determined by placing three fingers on the patient's wrist (left and right in turn). Information is also obtained by palpation, or tapping on different parts of the body, for example the abdomen, to detect accumulations of gas or liquid.

There is a popular belief that a good Chinese physician can know everything about a patient, including the detection of early pregnancy, by taking the patient's pulse. There are even stories of imperial physicians who took pulses by tying a string to their wrists and detecting pulse through the string without touching the patient, then went on to make an accurate diagnosis of the patient's condition. Legend has it that the empress and concubines of a Chinese emperor could not be physically touched by the physician who therefore had to rely on this unusually discreet method of pulse-taking. Needless to say, such methods remain legends.

It is true that experienced physicians often make quite accurate judgments of the patient's syndromes through pulse-taking, but the reality is that by the time he takes the pulse he has done some of the inspection and listening/olfaction of the four examinations. The ordinary physician would treat pulse-taking as just another dimension of information to be added to the other three. Although an important indicator, it need not be the most crucial one; neither is it normally sufficient to allow the physician to determine accurately the syndromes present in the patient. Nevertheless it cannot be denied that pulse-taking is a crucial part of the examination process for a patient.

Pulses are classified into more than 20 categories, taking into account texture, depth (how hard one needs to press with the

Table 6.3   Pulse Type and Indication.

Type of Pulse	Indication
Floating pulse浮脉	External syndrome, near skin level
Sunken pulse沉脉	Internal syndrome, deeper in the body
Moderately slow pulse缓脉	Dampness and weakness in spleen/stomach
Fast pulse数脉	Heat syndrome
Weak pulse虚脉	Asthenic syndrome, usually in *qi* and blood
Feeble pulse弱脉	Decline in *qi* and blood
Powerful pulse实脉	Sthenic syndrome
Slippery pulse滑脉	Retention of phlegm and fluid; sthenic heat
Thready pulse细脉	Asthenia of *qi* and blood
Taut pulse弦脉	Phlegm; liver and gall-bladder disorders
Tense pulse紧脉	Cold syndrome; food retention

fingers to feel it), and the perceived waveform. Some of the common pulses encountered in clinical practice and their usual indications are listed in Table 6.3.

6.2.3.2 *Therapeutic methods*

After a diagnosis is made and the syndromes differentiated, therapy, the second part of *bianzhenglunzhi* is applied. The principle involved is simple: treat a condition with opposing and balancing force, for example:

When there is heat, use cooling methods.

When there is cold, use warming methods.

When there is deficiency, tonify.

When there is excess, purge.

When there is impediment to *qi* flow, promote the flow of *qi*.

When there is blood stasis, 'liven' the blood flow and resolve the stasis.

When there is dampness, use diuresis and/or drying methods.

When there is wind, calm and extinguish it.

When there is phlegm, resolve it.

The application of therapeutic methods is mainly by the use of herbs, acupuncture and medical massage (*tuina* 推拿); they can each be used singly or in combination. The last method, *tuina*, may be used in place of acupuncture for patients (like children and the elderly) who cannot take acupuncture, or in place of herbs for those who cannot tolerate the side effects of some herbs.[161]

The Chinese pharmacopeia comprises thousands of materials of natural origin, inclusive of plant parts, minerals and animal parts (collectively known as *materia medica* or simply 'herbs'). There are also hundreds of complex formulations of these herbs to achieve therapeutic effects like cooling, warming, purging and tonification. For example, a patient who is diagnosed with the syndrome of a deficiency in kidney *yang* can be given *yang* tonics for the kidney such as cordyceps and *lurong* (deer horn). Heat syndromes can be cleared with a wide variety of herbs. The choice of herbs must take into account their effectiveness for heat in particular parts of the body: for example, *shigao* (gypsum) and *huangqin* (*radix scutellariae*) are commonly used for internal heat in the lung, *mudanpi* (the bark of the peony plant) for heat in the blood; *bohe* (peppermint) and *juhua* (chrysanthemum) for expelling heat at the superficies.

The proper use of herbs and herbal formulations is a large subject that incorporates several thousands of years of clinical experience and experimentation with their use. The theory of using of herbs and herbal formulations is an essential part of TCM theory, drawing on concepts from the other models like the meridian and organs systems, the eight rubrics, and the characteristics of entities like *qi*, blood, *jinye* (body fluids), dampness and wind.

---

[161] *Qigong* therapy, involving meditation and breathing exercises, is used in some circumstances, although some forms of *qigong* are shrouded in mystique and have possible spiritual or psychiatric dimensions. Most TCM physicians do not practise it.

The model of the five elements can be used to give the physician a wider repertoire of therapeutic options. If there is deficiency in one organ, the physician can choose to tonify the mother organ, as we observed earlier in the case of tonifying the spleen to strengthen the lung that suffers from a deficiency syndrome. For example, if lung-*qi* is in a state of deficiency, a tonic for the spleen-*qi* is deemed an effective remedy.

6.3 Epistemological Issues in TCM Models

As components of a scientific theory, TCM models must be able to explain physiological phenomena and the causes of illnesses. They must also be applicable to the diagnosis of illnesses and to the therapeutic methods used. They should be capable of making predictions that can be tested by experiments. Preferably there should also be descriptions of the underlying physical nature of TCM entities and how they can be detected, identified and measured.

The last point was addressed earlier in Chapters 4 and 5 on TCM entities, and organ and meridian systems. I suggested that some TCM entities are abstractions of underlying biochemical entities and processes, in effect theoretical constructs to fit TCM models of explanation and prediction. *Qi*, for example, is a generic term that can be a substance or a driving force for most physiological processes in the body, depending on the context of use. Some meanings of *qi* such air or breath can be identified and measured. The *qi* of an organ represents the ability of that organ to carry out its functions, as in spleen-*qi* for the digestive function. In principle, measures of the adequacy and level of spleen-*qi* can be devised based on biomedical indicators of how well the body is absorbing and converting nutrients to nourish the body. Organs in TCM are clusters of functions and not necessarily identified with particular somatic structures. As abstractions, many TCM entities like *jing* (essence) would not appear to lend themselves to detection and measurement, but their biomedical correlates, like a sonorous voice for strong pectoral-*qi*, could serve that purpose.

Historically, TCM theory for explaining physiological phenomena and illnesses evolved largely from the belief that the human body is a microcosm of the universe; hence truth in medicine should start from cosmology. This was the case with the *yin-yang* concept and the five-element model. In the case of the five-element model, Needham notes that it dates back to between 350 and 270 BC, to the time of the philosopher Tsou Yen, whom Needham regards as the "real founder of all Chinese scientific thought", although similar ideas had been in circulation for a hundred years or so before him. The *Shih Chi* (*Book of History*) records that Tsou Yen despaired over rulers becoming dissolute and lacking in virtue, and sought wisdom in the writing of the great sages. He invoked the cycles of *yin* and *yang* to classify natural phenomena and proposed the idea of the Five Powers (Virtues) that guide the course of history. Changes in history would be viewed as manifestations of changes at the lower inorganic levels of fire, wood, earth, water and earth. Every ruling house reigned only by virtue of one of the elements of the series.

Lloyd and Sivin point out that while the five elements show some superficial similarity to the four elements of Aristotle, there are really no counterparts in ancient Greek medicine. In their view, the term 'five elements' originated in the sphere of morality and became part of cosmological thought only in 240 AD.[162] In the Han dynasty (206 BC–220 AD), the five elements gradually came to be associated with every conceivable category — five

---

[162] Lloyd and Sivin (2002:259).

grains, five senses, five seasons (with the addition of the peak summer month) and, for physicians, the five *zang*-organs and their relationship to human emotions.

Although the historical origins of Chinese medical beliefs as contained in classics like the *Neijing* and the *Treatise on Febrile Diseases* are of interest primarily to the medical anthropologist, it is often used by detractors to attack TCM theory. This was one of the main points of the criticism in the 1920s and 1930s following the May 4th Movement of 1919.

The validity of models derived from or inspired by ancient beliefs should be assessed by the methods of science and not by the antiquity of their origins. The fact that the bear is a powerful animal may have influenced the choice of the bile of bears, rather than rabbits, to be used as medicine for the relief of high fevers.[163] There were, however, other strong animals available, like the wild boar, tigers and elephants. The Chinese pharmacopeia's settling for bear bile for certain types of fevers would be based on its perceived efficacy learned from clinical experience, after having tried out secretions from other animal sources. Animal parts are regularly used in folk medicine but most are not accepted in the Chinese pharmacopeia. For example, sorghum wine flavoured with a tiger penis immersed in it to enhance male potency does not appear in the Chinese pharmacopeia, no doubt because of its failure to deliver results. Unfortunately the tiger is being hunted to extinction for its bone and other body parts deemed by superstition and folk medicine to have medicinal value. Such beliefs have no place in TCM and do little for its scientific image.

Regardless of their origins, the models of TCM, whether derived from cosmology, folklore, or plain superstition, were

---

[163] This point was used by, a trained biochemist and a rabid critic of Chinese medicine, as an argument for concluding that Chinese medical theory and practice are superstitions.

subjected to test over time through the clinical work of physicians. They would have been refined, amended and expanded to best fit clinical experience. *Hence the prevailing ideology in TCM is that empirical observation should be the ultimate guide for medical theory.* In this sense, TCM is evidence-based medicine in a basic rudimentary form.

As a young researcher in Guangzhou in 1982, noted medical anthropologist Judith Farquhar innocuously asked how doctors knew which medical explanation was correct, and was cryptically told: "We take experience (*jingyan* 经验) to be our main guide and practice (*shijian* 实践) to be the main thing."[164] Such a response is in accord with the current pragmatic empiricism governing Chinese political and economic ideology, captured in the dictum: "*Gain truth from the facts*" (*shishi qiu shi* 实事求是). Deng Xiaoping, who launched the Chinese economic transformation from socialist central planning to a market economy in 1978, was the prime proponent of this philosophy, epitomized in a remark made during a state visit to Texas, "It does not matter if a cat is white or black as long as it catches mice." Such bold pragmatism has obvious implications for medical scientists obsessed with ontological issues of TCM entities and epistemic credentials of TCM models. In medical practice as least, the truth is what works.

6.3.1 *Heuristic models*

TCM practice uses heuristic empirical models which are the results of attempts to arrive at useful frameworks for explanation and prediction that translate into diagnosis and therapy. Diagnosis of symptoms allows them to be classified under patterns of illness or syndromes. Therapeutic methods predict that the administration of appropriate herbs and other therapeutic procedure like

---

[164] Farquhar (1994:1).

acupuncture and *tuina* would bring about relief from these symptoms.

The models are heuristic in the sense of being designed to best fit empirical experience. This is analogous to curve-fitting, drawing the best straight or curved line through a set of observations plotted on a two-dimensional graph. After the curve is drawn, one finds a mathematical formula to best describe the curve over a relevant range. The formula could be as simple as a straight line a+bx, a quadratic function $a+bx+cx^2$, or one of an infinite number of other more complicated functions. The starting curve fit is often a straight line; a more sophisticated one could involve exponential, logarithmic and more complex functions with boundary conditions. TCM models are like straight lines, often crude and lacking in accuracy but modified and refined over time to better fit clinical situations encountered over the history of Chinese medicine.

The analogy of the black box in cybernetics may also be helpful. Observers cannot see what is in the box but are able to measure its external manifestations. By measuring inputs and outputs, one makes conjectures about what is in the box and tries to find the mathematical equation that best relates output to input.[165]

Some orthodox Chinese medical thinkers do not necessarily subscribe to this empiricist view of TCM models, believing that the ancients had divine visions and were able to relate cosmological models to those of the human body. An important part of the working of these visions was the ability, through introspection, to gain understanding of the inner workings of one's body.[166] There is no reason to believe that introspection has such epistemic powers, or that the ancients had special insights other than those

---

[165] Huang (1995:18–21) discusses this analogy in some depth.
[166] See Liu Lihong (2003:14–16).

gained by ordinary mortals using reasoning and conjecture and appealing to the weight of clinical evidence from medical practice. Admittedly, a large proportion of practising TCM physicians is orthodox; most of them may not agree with my view of the heuristic nature of TCM models.

6.4 Reductionism, Holism and Systems Biology

In recent years, the TCM model of syndrome differentiation, which plays a central role in TCM theory, may have indirectly gained support from attempts to apply the approach of the emergent science of systems biology to biomedical research.

Systems biology focuses on complex interactions within biological systems, making claims to the use of a holistic rather than a reductionist perspective of biomedical processes. A principal aim is to model properties of cells and tissues functioning as a system that involves metabolic networks and cell signalling networks. The study of the interactions between the building blocks of biological systems and the implications of interactions for the proper functioning of the system is believed to constitute a more complete paradigm that overcomes the shortcomings of reductionism. Sauer puts it as follows:

> The reductionist approach has successfully identified most of the components and many of the interactions but, unfortunately, offers no convincing concepts or methods to understand how system properties emerge . . . the pluralism of causes and effects in biological networks is better addressed by observing, through quantitative measures, multiple components simultaneously and by rigorous data integration with mathematical model[s].[167]

---

[167] Sauer *et al.* (2007:550–551).

Systems biology strikes a consonant chord with TCM researchers in China who have held in awe the progress of molecular and cellular biology and the consequent focus swing of biomedical science to the cellular and genomic level, but at the same time held serious reservations over the ability of a reductionist approach to medicine in modelling the complexity of the human body. Zhu, for example, points that the presentation of the body in terms of the molecular structure of cells and genes omits the relationships that hold these units together to function as a biological system.[168] More recently Leroy Hood, president of the Institute for Systems Biology, offered a point of view that appears to echo TCM holism with advocacy of 4P health care (predictive, personalised, preventive and participatory). This focuses on the biochemical networks underlying health and disease, then aims to treat and prevent disease by identifying and countering perturbations in the biological networks.[169] For example, researchers led by Jia used phenotyping technologies to simultaneously characterise multiple drug responses to dietary preparations, such as the health tea *pu-er*, by measuring the absorption of tea molecules, the output of gut bacteria metabolism, and the human metabolic response profile in the urine. Phenotyping strategy, they argue, can further differentiate disease subtypes that are correlated to different TCM syndromes.[170]

The systems biology approach to medicine nurtures hope for a partial convergence of TCM and Western medicine by identifying biomedical phenomena that correlate with TCM entities and models. While there is some potential in this approach, the

---

[168] Zhu (2005).

[169] Peng (2011).

[170] These findings of a research team led by Jia are reported in Peng (2011), based on Xie *et al.* (2009). Characterization of Pu-erh Tea Using Chemical and Metabolic Profiling Approaches *Journal of Agricultural and Food Chemistry* 57: 3046–3054.

challenge will be in the details. It may be doomed to failure if, as I shall argue later,[171] there may not exist a unique set of biomarkers for each particular syndrome; this is akin to the concept of multiple realisation in the philosophy of science.[172]

For system biology methods to apply to TCM theory, there also needs to be an understanding of the epistemic status of TCM entities like *qi*, wind and phlegm and an appreciation of the heuristic nature of TCM models, so that one does not embark on the futile task of finding a one-to-one correspondence between TCM theory and biomedical laws and regularities.

6.5 The Nature of TCM Models: Summing Up

The model of therapy based on syndrome differentiation classifies constellations of symptoms into categories of excess, deficiency, heat, coldness, obstructed flow and also into sub-categories depending on the locus of the pathology (for example, '*yin* deficiency of the kidney'). Such classifications allow illness patterns, or syndromes, to be identified by diagnosis. Therapeutic methods are then applied in accordance with the syndromes thus differentiated, for example applying cooling methods to heat syndromes and tonification for deficiency syndromes.

That these therapeutic models are testable, and indeed should be tested if TCM is to make scientific claims, is a key conclusion of this book, to be presented in Chapter 7.

---

[171] Chapter 7.
[172] See, for example, Okasha (2002:56–57).

Chapter 7

Evidence for TCM Theory

The notion that evidence can be reliably placed in hierarchies is illusory.
Hierarchies place RCTs on an undeserved pedestal.

Sir Michael Rawlins

Evidence for TCM theory can broadly be divided into two categories:

(a) Evidence for the existence of TCM entities and the detection/ measurement of their properties;
(b) Evidence for the usefulness and efficacy of TCM diagnostic and therapeutic methods.

With regard to the first category, I have argued that TCM entities are a motley collection of observable biochemical substances like blood and body fluids, as well as abstractions and theoretical constructs (*qi, jing,* wind, organs, meridians, etc.) representing underlying biochemical entities and processes to fit TCM heuristic models. Viewed in this way, seeking direct evidence for the existence of a TCM entity is not a sensible enterprise.

The second category, evidence for TCM models in explanation and prediction, should be the core of any enquiry into the scientific usefulness and validity of TCM theory. TCM does not provide explanations in the reductionist terms of biomedical science. It does not explain the behaviour of such entities as *qi* and phlegm using knowledge in molecular biology. Nor does it reduce these to those found in the physical sciences, notwithstanding various innovative if bizarre efforts to do so; for example, the attempt by some modern physicists to interpret entities like *qi* in terms of quantum theory.[173]

TCM models do attempt to provide explanations for illnesses and their progression into various syndromes, and prescribe treatment according to syndrome diagnosis. *These treatments are in principle testable and should form the focus of investigations into the validity of TCM models.*

Before discussing methods of finding evidence for the TCM models of therapy, it is necessary first to dispose of the epistemological contention that TCM is a different Kuhnian paradigm from Western biomedicine and therefore should not be subjected to the same testing methods of evidence-based medicine.

7.1 TCM as Evidence-Based Medicine

Arguing for Chinese medicine to be a different paradigm from biomedical medicine, Fan asserts:

> The philosophy of science has convincingly shown that between two incommensurable, competing theoretical systems (such as the theoretical systems of traditional Chinese medicine and modern scientific medicine), it is only begging the question or making a circular argument to claim that one is more true than the other...the Chinese should change their monostandard integration to a dual standard integration, where modern scientific medicine will be practiced and developed according to the modern scientific standard, and traditional Chinese medicine will be allowed to practice and develop in terms of its own standard.[174]

---

[173] See, for example, Lo (2004).
[174] Fan (2003:218–219).

Along the same vein, Churchill contends that

> Many scientists believe that the scientific paradigm has absolute
> truth value, but philosophers such as Thomas Kuhn reject this. If no
> paradigm does have absolute value, there is no absolute basis with
> which to judge another paradigm. Any paradigm will appear limited
> or incorrect from the perspective of a different paradigm, so Chinese
> medicine will seem incorrect from a biomedical point of view.[175]

Putting aside the dubious interpretation of Kuhn in both
instances, it takes an epistemological leap to go from the assertion —
that two systems of medicine belong to two different (scientific)
paradigms — to the contention that the methods of evidence-based
medicine used in one does not therefore apply to the other. Granted
that the differentiation of syndromes in TCM is distinctive to
Chinese medicine and not used in Western medicine, why should it
follow that TCM methods are absolved from clinical tests to establish their usefulness and validity? To use a trite analogy, if two religions worship different gods, it does not follow that followers of
both religions cannot use the same evangelical methods for winning
over non-believers.

The only escape from evidence-based medicine is to take the
view that evidence-based science is itself a Western paradigm and
not a traditional Chinese one, and therefore not applicable to truth
in Chinese medicine. Such an ideological position is tantamount

---

[175]Churchill (1999:33). In a *British Medical Journal* paper, Tang (2006) takes a more
eclectic position, conceding that Chinese and Western medicines may belong to two
different "paradigms" but that does not rule out each having theories that are testable
by the conventional methods of science found in evidence-based medicine. I am in
agreement with this approach, except that as explained earlier, I do not take the view
they belong to two different paradigms (in Kuhn's sense of disciplinary matrix) but
that they have some paradigms (exemplars) in common and others that are different.
See Kuhn (1974) for a redefinition of paradigms.

to rejecting conventional wisdom that the scientific experiment is, as Krauss puts it, "the ultimate arbiter of truth" about the world.[176] It is a difficult position to defend. As I shall argue below, it is not even necessary to adhere to this position just to avoid subjecting Chinese medicine to those protocols of evidence-based medicine that were devised to test and approve Western drugs for mass-market consumption. Chinese medical interventions can be subjected to the rigours of evidence-based medicine, but using protocols suited to the way these interventions are applied.

However, on the claim that truths about the mortal and material world should be subjected to scientific experimentation, we should in fairness recognise that there is a case for alternative ideologies. The counter argument to the scientific experimentation ideology is that science itself cannot prove the proposition that all truths about the world should be established by its methods. In other words, the theory "Science is the only path to truth" is itself not capable of proof by experimentation. A similar argument has been adduced, with devastating effect, against Karl Popper's falsifiability criterion for scientific theory (that a theory is not scientific if it cannot be falsified).

Truth in Chinese medicine — the ancient Chinese thinkers believed and traditionalists accept — can also be obtained by *introspection* or what one could interpret as "spiritual discernment".[177] Acceptance of either the scientific method or the spiritual discernment alternative each requires a leap of faith. Interestingly, in advocating a more pluralistic view of avenues to truth, the distinguished medical anthropologist Arthur Kleinman postulates that monotheism in the Western tradition has had a determinative effect on biomedicine: the idea of a single god legitimates the idea

---

[176] Krauss (2012).

[177] See, for example, Liu (2003) whose views were summarised in Chapter 2.

of a single underlying truth and destroys tolerance for alternative paradigms.[178] That scientific experimentation is the only path to truth is one such paradigm. The claim that only the reductionist methods of biomedicine can explain disease and its cure could be viewed as consequence of this monotheistic mindset.

The ideological position that Chinese and Western medicines belong to two incommensurable paradigms — one based on science, and the other based on a separate path to knowledge (discernment) — has a small but significant scholarly following among traditionalists. Be that as it may, an objective of this book is to ascertain how TCM can be understood by modern science and, if it wishes to gain acceptance by scientists for some its therapies, how the methods of evidence-based medicine may be applied to it. The traditionalist argument, while appealling to a large number of TCM researchers who are well-versed in modern science, but not willing grant it exclusive access to truth, cannot help Western science understand and accept those parts of TCM, if any, that can be shown to be efficacious by outcome measures of clinical trials. It is therefore more useful to keep our focus on how TCM therapies can be subjected to the testing methods of evidence-based medicine.

7.2 Clinical Trials on TCM Therapies

The key model to test is that of therapy based on syndrome differentiation, from which hypotheses concerning appropriate therapies to be applied are derived and testable by the hypothetico-deductive method.

It is first necessary to differentiate between two kinds of clinical trials for therapies that have been attributed to Chinese medicine:

---

[178] Kleinman (1995).

a. Clinical trials on herbs or combinations of herbs for specific (Western) diseases, and of acupuncture for relief of pain or specific symptoms like pain and dizziness. Examples are the use of the herb *danshen (salvia miltiorrhiza)* for ischemic coronary heart disease and acupuncture at points on the head, face and hands for migraine headaches.

b. Clinical trials on the use of herbs and herbal formulations, or acupuncture points, for treating TCM syndromes. Examples would be the use of *Liuwei Dihuang Wan* for treatment of the syndrome of deficiency in kidney *yin*, and a combination of acupuncture points along the spleen stomach meridians to treat syndromes of weakness in spleen-*qi* and dampness in the spleen.

7.2.1 *Clinical trials on western herbal medicine and western acupuncture*

The first category is best viewed as trials of Western medicine's methods of therapy using materials and techniques borrowed from Chinese medical sources. These trials are part of the process of developing new drugs from Chinese sources and of validating acupuncture procedures for therapeutic purposes.

Traditionally, drugs in the West were discovered by identifying the active ingredient from traditional remedies and occasionally by serendipitous discovery.[179] With advances in the knowledge of disease and infection at the molecular levels, scientists now more commonly try to find compounds that specifically modulate those molecules and thereby design new drugs. Such drug discovery processes, whether by traditional methods or by modern methods of design, involve the identification of candidates

---

[179] Serendipitous discovery occurs when one finds a cure for a disease while looking for a cure for another. See, for example, Ban (2006:335–344).

and their characterisation, screening, and assays for therapeutic efficacy. Once a substance has shown its value in these tests, the process of drug development proceeds to clinical trials. Chinese herbal medications provide a potentially rich source of drug discovery from traditional natural sources.

Clinical trials on herbal medications have been carried out mainly by Western researchers in Europe, North America and Australia, and increasingly in China as well. These trials are conducted on the raw herbs as well as extracts. They typically follow the protocol and meet the standards of rigour for evidence-based medicine to varying extents. Most of them use randomised controlled trials (RCTs), treating a Chinese herb, or a prescription consisting of a number of herbs, like a Western drug or a cocktail of drugs.

Such trials should be viewed as testing the efficacy of Chinese herbs used like Western drugs to relieve symptoms or treat disease. In more advanced stages of drug discovery, chemical constituents of the herbs are found that have the desired therapeutic effect. These are then extracted and made into the active ingredients for regular Western drugs (or synthesised so that the herb is redundant). Examples are *Ginko bilova*, an extract of the ginko leaf, now prescribed by Western doctors for improving blood circulation in the brain, and *Crataegutt*, an extract of the hawthorne leaves and flowers, used to promote coronary and myocardial blood flow and improve the oxygen utilization of the heart. Both were developed in German pharmaceutical laboratories. Of course many Western cardiac remedies like aspirin and digitalis also come from natural sources other than those of Chinese medicine.

Trials of such Chinese herbal medications and their subsequent development and adoption as Western drugs lend credence to the notion that Chinese herbs have medicinal value, but *such trials do not in themselves directly validate TCM theory.* The drugs discovered in this way make a contribution to the pharmaceutical industry's role of providing new and better modern drugs. But they do not endorse the practice of Chinese medicine any more than the use of quinine, an extract of a bark used by South American natives to treat malaria, is a validation of South American native medical theory. For convenience we term drugs developed by pharmaceutical firms using herbs or herb extracts for the treatment of specific diseases or symptoms as parts of 'Western herbal medicine'.

Likewise, trials on acupuncture points for symptomatic relief of pain and dizziness are validations of 'Western acupuncture'. Where these trials suggest the efficacy of these acupuncture methods, biomedical explanations are usually sought by researchers for physiological responses of the body to needling.[180] These explanations do not necessarily support or even relate to the TCM meridian system that forms the basis of the selection of TCM acupuncture points for treatment of specific conditions. To test TCM acupuncture theory, one needs to investigate if it produces better results than Western acupuncture not based on the Chinese meridian system, or is better than 'sham acupuncture' (when needles are inserted in the wrong places or only appear to the patient to have been inserted).

7.2.2 *Clinical trials on TCM treatment of TCM syndromes*

The second category of clinical trials tests hypotheses on TCM methods of treatment based on the differentiation of syndromes. Such trials have yet to be carried out to any significant extent. I

---

[180] See, for example, various papers in the volume by Ernst and White (1999).

propose with two examples below how they may be carried out using the classical hypothetico-deductive method.

Example 1: Patients with a constellation of symptoms P are diagnosed with syndrome S and are treated by therapy method T which TCM prescribes based on the principle of syndrome differentiation and corresponding treatment.

> **Main Hypothesis:** Syndrome S can be treated by use of therapy method T
>
> Initial Condition: The patient exhibits the set of symptoms P
>
> Initial Condition: Syndrome S is identified ('differentiated') through TCM diagnosis of symptoms P
>
> ---
>
> **Observational Prediction:** Applying therapy T results in a reduction in the symptoms P in the patient

An example of syndrome S would be deficiency of kidney-*yin* which is identified ('differentiated') by a physician as a constellation of symptoms that includes aching and weakness of the loins and knees, dizziness and tinnitus, night sweats, dry mouth and throat, afternoon flush in the cheeks, insomnia, thin rapid pulse, and a red tongue with little fur.[181] A tonic pill like *Liuwei Dihuang Wan* 六味地黄丸 ('pill of six ingredients with *rehmanniae*') is used for two weeks on a randomised sample of patients, with a control group offered placebo pills of the same appearance and similar taste. If there is a significant difference in the improvement of the symptoms of the first group compared to those of the second, the main hypothesis is confirmed.

---

[181] See, for example, Wang (2002:234).

Example 2: The five-element model is used together with the method of syndrome differentiation and treatment for patients with a constellation of symptoms P

> **Main Hypothesis:** Syndrome S in organ C can be treated by use of tonic therapy T for the mother organ M
>
> Auxiliary Hypothesis: Tonic for the mother organ helps the child organ (applying the five-element model)
>
> Initial Condition: The patient exhibits symptoms P
>
> Initial Condition: Symptoms P are differentiated as syndrome S in organ C
>
> ───────────────────────────────────
>
> **Observational Prediction:** Applying therapy T to the mother organ M heals syndrome S in the child organ C

Syndrome S could be deficiency in lung-*qi* differentiated by the method of the four examinations. The prescribed therapy T consists of treating the mother organ M (spleen) with a spleen-*qi* tonic such as *Sijunzi Tang* 四君子汤 ('Decoction of the Four Noble Herbs').

The two examples above could in principle be the subjects of double-blind RCTs. Patients and physicians employed to conduct syndrome differentiation would be blinded with regard to which patients received the treatment T and which received a placebo. There are however potential methodological challenges in conducting such trials.

1. Syndromes are in a dynamic state, hence for practical purposes clinical trials should be limited to those syndromes that are relatively stable and that do not change without intervention within the duration of the trial. For example, most cases of

deficiency of kidney-*yin* tend to be chronic, accompanying age-ing and prolonged stress; prolonged weakened kidney-*yin* also frequently occurs for patients who have recovered from severe fevers and infections, or have received strong Western treat-ments like chemotherapy and radiation therapy. TCM treat-ments that claim to be able to resolve this condition may take many weeks or months, hence these cases would be suitable for RCTs carried out over a relatively long trial periods. But there are also cases of kidney-*yin* being damaged with inadequate sleep and stress. Most of these are claimed by TCM to resolve within a week or two with suitable medication, hence a RCT spread over about a week would be an appropriate test for this TCM claim. An appropriate refinement of the clinical trials would employ samples of people that belong to the first cate-gory (chronic cases) or the other (shorter-term cases), but not a mixture of the two. This would naturally reduce the sample sizes available.

2. Patients often have more than one syndrome present. For example, patients with kidney-*yang* deficiency may also have weakness in spleen-*qi*. Some of the ingredients commonly used in prescriptions for kidney-*yang* deficiency have the side effect of helping with spleen-*qi*. The result is that there may be an improvement in the symptoms of both syndromes, and as some of these symptoms are shared by these syn-dromes, the actual effect of the prescription on the main syndrome would be difficult to isolate.

3. The physician's diagnosis based on 'the four examinations' described in the last chapter is the standard method for determining the presence of a syndrome. This is subject to human error and erroneous judgment as the complex mix-ture of symptoms when there is more than one syndrome present can make differentiation of syndromes trickier and

require more highly-skilled and experienced physicians. When multiple syndromes are present, the physician sees a basket of symptoms from which he has to sort out several constellations, each corresponding to a syndrome. With many of the syndromes having one or more symptoms in common, like a rapid pulse or a pale tongue, there may be more than one permutation of syndromes to produce the same basket of symptoms. (The complex basket of symptoms could be multiply-realised at the level of underlying syndromes.) Sometimes the symptoms are hard to determine, for example the colour of the face and tongue, which are already different across individuals in healthy states: a pale face may be healthy for one with a fair complexion but sickly for one with a ruddy complexion. Hence, it is possible for experienced physicians to disagree on the syndromes when they observe the same symptoms. A similar situation exists with the diagnosis of, for example, clinical depression in Western psychiatry. A patient is deemed to have depression if he has more than an arbitrarily fixed number of symptoms. In practice, psychiatrists can differ on the diagnosis after observing the same patient, even if there was no disagreement on the symptoms observed, and divergence of opinion was only on the interpretation of the symptoms. But such situations are much less common in Western medicine than in TCM.[182]

---

[182] For animal studies in which the application of the four examinations is not feasible, Lu *et al.* (2009:501–505) propose the method of determining the presence of a syndrome by observing the animal responses to a standard Chinese herb prescription for that syndrome: those that respond are then deemed to have the syndrome, and biological biomarkers of these are then studied compared to those that do not respond. Such a methodology presumes that the efficacy of the prescription for that syndrome, something that needs to be separately established.

These methodological problems are not peculiar to TCM, but tend to be more troublesome with TCM therapies. Clinical trials for Western medical treatments also face problems of unstable disease symptoms and multiple diseases in the same person, but the problems are more challenging for TCM clinical trials because TCM syndromes are of a more dynamic nature, generally changing at a faster rate than conditions classified as diseases in Western medicine.

It should be noted that when we speak of TCM syndromes being of a more dynamic nature, we refer to the syndromes as *differentiated* (identified) by the methods of TCM diagnosis for which a particular constellation of symptoms defines the syndrome. Hence perceived dynamism is a matter of observation of changing symptoms.

TCM physicians are also accustomed to providing individualised treatment, adjusting the dosage and composition of medication to the person's constitution, the severity of his symptoms and the appearance of other syndromes as his condition evolves. This contrasts with Western medicine, which tends to stay with a fixed dosage of single-ingredient medication over a prolonged period of the patient's disease. For example, a person with early chronic Type II diabetes is prescribed the drug Metformin (500 mg twice daily) to control blood sugar level, taken over a period of months or years. A Chinese physician treating the same condition (with herbal medications rather than Metformin) watches the syndromes of the patient such as *yin* deficiency of the lung; this causes thirstiness and frequent urination and *qi* stagnation of the liver, which is accompanied by vexatious moods. He is likely to modify the prescription, comprising a cocktail of herbs, every one or two weeks in accordance with the patient's evolving syndromes at each visit. If lung-*yin* deficiency has improved but liver-*qi* stagnation has not, the physician might reduce the dosage of those herbs that address *yin* deficiency and increase it for herbs that treat *qi* stagnation. Using RCTs to test TCM treatment constrains the physician to one prescription for all patients in the treatment arm, resulting in what the TCM physician would deem to be compromised efficacy of the treatment.

Hence the argument could be made that the conventional protocol of RCTs constrains the efficacy of TCM treatments to be tested, and is therefore biased against the validation of the true efficacy of TCM therapies. Conceivably, however, the protocol could be modified for periodic diagnosis by physicians of patients in both the treatment and control arms of the trial and suitable changes in the prescription for the treatment arm patients (and change to the appearance of the placebo given to the control arm patients.) But physicians would perforce no longer be blinded.

The problem of human error arising from the key role of the diagnosing physician applying the four examinations is a more troublesome one. One could with justice make the counter argument that diagnostic error is also perfectly possible in the Western approach. However it should be recognised that with a large arsenal of diagnostic tools from blood tests to CT scans and separate professional expertise for reading and interpreting test results for the physician, Western diagnosis leaves less room for human error. One could interpret this as indicating that Western diagnosis is more scientific; it could certainly claim to be more objective because of the lower risk of human error.

7.2.3 Biomarkers

Although there is in practice a high degree of consistency in the diagnosis of common syndromes by TCM physicians, this would not be the case for multiple syndromes. If there were established biomarkers for determining the presence of any particular syndrome, this would greatly simplify the problem, but to date, the use of biomarkers for differentiating syndromes has not been satisfactorily achieved. Some researchers have tried using statistical data mining methods to develop these biomarkers.[183] Such methods are not without problems.

The use of biomarkers makes the presumption that there is an exact set of biological states, such as the presence of microbiological pathogens or changes in the level of blood component or endocrinal secretions, corresponding to a TCM syndrome. But is every syndrome associated with a unique set of biomarkers? There is no reason to believe that this would in fact be the case of all syndromes, or even any syndrome. There is a similar issue in Western medicine for more complex conditions like rheumatoid arthritis, for which the RA (rheumatoid arthritis) factor measured from blood samples is used as a probabilistic indicator of the presence of the disease, but the correlation is notoriously imperfect. A person with a high RA factor may have no symptoms (false positive), and an acute rheumatoid arthritis sufferer exhibiting classical symptoms of inflamed joints and connective tissue may have a normal RA factor (false negative). Recent research findings indicate that the PSA index used for detection of prostate cancer is similarly flawed.[184] For most diseases in biomedicine, however, the biomarkers are unambiguous. For example the presence of lung lesions seen in chest X-rays and the presence of the *tubercle bacillus* in the blood is a definitive indicator of tuberculosis, or the presence of the rhinovirus in blood and nasal discharges a definitive indicator of the common cold.

In the case of TCM syndromes, no accepted set of biomarkers has been established for any syndrome. The nature of TCM

---

[183] Guo *et al.* (2009:531–546).
[184] Damber and Aus (2008).

syndromes may well be such that finding a unique set of biomarkers for each syndrome is not feasible. Interestingly, some of the conditions for which Western medicine uses the term 'syndrome' are also difficult to pin down consistently with biomarkers, for example chronic fatigue and irritable bowel syndromes. This may well be the reason that the same English term 'syndrome' has been chosen for the translation of the TCM term *'zheng'* (证).

The fact that most diseases recorded in Western medicine have clear and unambiguous biomarkers whereas TCM syndromes are (at least currently) totally lacking in biomarkers could subject TCM to the charge that TCM is unscientific and merely hiding behind subtlety and complexity to account for lack of supporting evidence. The emphasis on biomarkers follows from a reductionist approach to medicine, an approach that modern TCM physicians readily concede has many advantages over ancient Chinese methods of diagnosis. But these same physicians would argue that medicine is not necessarily entirely reducible to biomedical parameters, nor are the methods of biomedicine the only or even always the best route to achieving effective therapy. Such a defence of TCM can be and indeed is often made, and it leaves open the question of which method of diagnosis yields better information for prescribing therapies. While Western diagnosis has a proven record of providing reliable information on which suitable therapeutic interventions may be prescribed, this is not the case with TCM. For TCM the priority for achieving credibility in the scientific realm remains that of providing evidence through clinical trials that it has therapeutic capabilities.

7.2.4 *Suitability of RCTs for TCM*

With the objective of bringing about better acceptance of TCM in mind, some researchers are prepared to accept the principles of evidence-based medicine but are convinced that, as the core of

TCM therapeutic method, the differentiation and treatment of syndromes cannot be subjected to RCTs. Shea (2006) summarises their views as follows:

> Discussions of the difficulty of applying the RCT design to Chinese medicine stress that while biomedicine assigns standardised treatment based on disease categories such as diabetes, Chinese medicine tailors individualised treatment based on syndromes[...]. RCT detractors assert that it is impossible to conduct valid RCTs on Chinese medicine because if syndrome differentiation was used, its radical individualisation would result in small numbers in the same treatment group, yielding results lacking statistical significance. Yet, if, to avoid the N=1 problem, Chinese medicine treatments were tested within a biomedical diagnostic framework, the results would be equally meaningless because Chinese medicine's fundamental essence would be violated.[185]

By ruling out RCTs for all clinical trials of TCM therapies, 'RCT detractors' run the risk of being dismissed by 'TCM detractors' who would charge that since TCM cannot be subjected to RCTs it is therefore not scientific. Either polar position leans toward the dogmatic and is at variance with the more enlightened views and cogent arguments offered by Urbach, Worrall, Rawlins and others that RCTs are not the only useful means for validating the efficacy of interventions; in fact oftentimes they are neither the best means nor even a feasible way of testing.[186] As Rawlins puts it, "the notion that evidence can be reliably placed in hierarchies is illusory" and such hierarchies with RCTs at their summit and various forms of observational studies "nestling in the foothills" put RCTs on an "undeserved pedestal".[187]

---

[185] Shea, JL (2006:258).
[186] Urbach (1985), Worrall (2002, 2007), Rawlins (2008).
[187] Rawlins (2008:1–2).

I think "RCT detractors" among TCM researchers are correct to de-emphasise RCTs but are being overly pessimistic to rule them out in all situations. While RCTs need not be the only way to conduct clinical trials and while there are considerable methodological difficulties dealing with syndromes for clinical trials as pointed out above, they can in principle be conducted when available samples are large enough. They do not violate any "fundamental essence" of TCM if the trials were conducted on differentiated syndromes and therapies applied according to TCM principles rather than on "Western herbal medicine" and "Western acupuncture".

TCM does emphasise individualised treatment by virtue of focusing on multiple syndromes in a dynamic state, which makes each patient potentially different from most others. This militates against the use of RCTs. But it can be argued that patients are all different anyway, whether looked at from the point of view of TCM or Western medicine. It is for RCTs to be designed in such a manner as to average out these differences such that the patient samples in the treatment and control arms of the RCTs are statistically as close as possible. This may not always be possible, which is why observational studies and case studies (covered further below) should also be considered and used when appropriate.

In sum, clinical trials based on syndrome differentiation tend to be more difficult compared to those for Western medicine, largely because of the highly patient-centric approach of TCM therapy. In practice, no two persons suffering from the same disease are likely to be given the same prescription by a TCM physician, in part because they have different constitutions but largely also because they are at different stages of the evolution of the illness and exhibit different syndromes in a dynamic state. Though not valid as a defence for the paucity and relatively poor quality of testing TCM theory through clinical trials, this suggests that alternative avenues for seeking evidence in TCM should also be actively investigated; particularly observational trials based on properly recorded patient data such as those now available in modern TCM hospitals in China. This is the most likely source of significant evidence supporting or invalidating TCM based on therapies administered to large number of patients in modern times, and it is a pressing area for future research.

7.2.5 Recent clinical trials

In recent years there have been a number of preliminary studies on the treatment of syndromes by TCM methods. Their findings are tentative and their methodologies leave much to be desired, leaving room for more and better research.[188] In effect, no rigorous clinical trials have been conducted (that I am aware of) on TCM therapies based solely on differentiation of syndromes.[189] There are two possible reasons for this.

First, the methodological difficulties that I outlined above have not yet been effectively addressed, leading to the phenomenon of 'RCT detractors' cited earlier.

Second, at a more fundamental level, TCM researchers are driven by the more practical objective of showing that Chinese medications can heal disease and acupuncture can provide symptomatic relief (mainly of pain). Success in such clinical trials draws attention from the medical community and opens up opportunities for drug discovery by Western pharmaceutical companies. From the point of these researchers, TCM theory guides them toward the particular acupuncture or herbal interventions to treat a disease (by addressing the syndromes commonly associated with that disease, e.g. weak spleen-*qi* for

---

[188]Lu *et al.* (2009), Zhang Jie (2005).
[189]One attempt was by Zheng (1985).

gastritis). Few feel motivated to convince Western science of the validity of TCM theory by focusing on syndrome differentiation and therapy. Like the late Chinese leader Deng Xiaoping, they are more concerned to show that the medicine works rather than to validate a particular theory explaining why it works.

Hence it is not surprising that nearly all clinical trials on Chinese medications and acupuncture points have been in the categories of Western herbal medicine and Western acupuncture. For example, in the 2010 international meeting of the Consortium for the Globalisation of Chinese Medicine (a multinational East-West organisation), over 300 papers covered clinical trials; among these fewer than 10 were in the category of testing TCM therapies, and even those dwelt mainly on unresolved methodological issues.[190] From the point of view of validating TCM theories clinical trials syndrome differentiation and treatment need to be conducted.

But even for clinical trials on Chinese medications and acupuncture for the treatment of diseases defined by Western medicine, the quality of work has not generally been satisfactory. Several Western researchers have conducted meta-analyses for trials for TCM treatments and concluded that the results are patchy, suggesting that certain conditions respond to TCM treatments but most others were either negative or likely placebo responses.[191] In general, research at Chinese and other East Asian universities tend to validate the efficacy of TCM treatments, while those carried out by Western researchers are largely negative. At the same time, it has been pointed that the standard of scientific rigour in the Eastern studies did not meet Western standards. Lai, a medical statistician at the Guangdong University

---

[190] A summary of such papers is presented in Bian (2010).TCM concepts in the trials, CGCM August 2010 presentation. The same pattern was seen in the 2011 meeting.
[191] See, for example, Tang *et al.*(1999) and Kaptchuk (2000:Appendix E).

of Chinese Medicine, conducted a meta-analysis of clinical trials in China on Western herbal therapies as well as TCM therapies and found most of them inadequate in methodological rigour.[192] A recent study by Shang *et al.* was only slightly more positive, concluding that the clinical evidence for the efficacy of Chinese medicine had "yet to be rigorously established".[193]

7.3 Observational Trials and Medical Case Studies

Given that evidence-based medicine is considered by some to have begun only in the 1950s with the advent of RCTs, one might ask as Worrall famously did: What on earth was medicine based on before?[194]

The answer seems obvious. Modern medicine has always been based on evidence, long before the RCT was invented and later zealously anointed as the gold standard for evidence. There have always been observational studies for Western medicine, and case studies, mostly, for Chinese medicine. Where case studies have been properly recorded and the information contained therein lends itself to statistical studies, they can form the database for observational studies.

7.3.1 *Evidence from case studies*

The use of cases as an analytical and pedagogical tool was institutionalised at Harvard Law School in the 19th century and over a hundred years ago at Harvard Business School. Case-based reasoning versus rule-based reasoning has been a subject of discussion in the recent philosophical literature.

---

[192] Lai (2001, 2010).

[193] Shang *et al.* (2007).

[194] Worrall (2002).

7.3.1.1 *Case-based reasoning*

Case-based reasoning does not attempt to solve a problem from first principles or a set of accepted rules or laws, as a rule-based system would. Instead, as Nickles argues, it employs "some sort of similarity metric to find one or more cases similar to the presented case" in attempting to find a resolution to a problem at hand.[195] Case-reasoning is not among Hacking's six modes of human reasoning: postulation and deduction, experimental exploration, construction of models by analogy, ordering of variety by comparison and taxonomy, statistical analysis of regularities, and historical derivation of genetic development, but one could argue that it should be added to the list.[196]

Case-based reasoning is an alternative to rule-based reasoning as exemplified by, for example, the hypothetico-deductive method. Instead of solving each new problem starting from some set of fundamental rules, we match the new problem to one or more problems and solutions sets already available in case archives. Instead of trying to solve a problem by applying some abstract rule, appeal is made to the contextually rich practical problems of the past. Routine or near-identical problems can be solved immediately, and less routine ones require judgment to combine previous cases in such a manner as to get a suitable fit with the new problem.

Critics of case-based reasoning could argue that such reasoning does not really eschew rules but simply conceals them by incorporating them in "the abstraction procedures and the corresponding indexing and retrieval mechanisms".[197] In other words, there is some hidden adherence to underlying rules in the

---

[195] Nickles (1998:70).
[196] Hacking (1992:2) and Forrester (1996).
[197] Nickles (2003:162).

way the relevant cases are selected for reference and applied. The classic Johnson and Johnson case at Harvard Business School involved the chief executive of the company taking the tough decision to make a nation-wide recall of Tylenol tablets that had been criminally laced with arsenic. It was a costly decision for what appeared to be only a very minor number of Tylenol tablets so affected, but it restored confidence in the company, whose public image subsequently soared together with its profitability. Certain rules emerged that can be used for dealing with future recall cases: accept responsibility, come clean with the media. Several decades later, the motor industry giant Toyota, to ever-lasting regret, did not heed these injunctions, and suffered per-manent damage to its reputation following a recall crisis in 2010 caused by a faulty accelerator pedal.

That cases have hidden rules does not however reduce the case to a set of rules because of the rich and complex context of business situations. This non-reducibility to a set of rules means that there will not normally be a correct or standard solution to a case, as there is in solving a problem in mechanics or chemistry. If another case of the Johnson and Johnson genre were to occur, the extent to which responsibility should be accepted and how the media should be handled are not reducible to rules but requires active management by a visionary and decisive CEO, using the past case as a guide but adding his judgment of the present context and complications to decide on a solution. The past case thus gives clues to similar approaches and methodolo-gies to use rather than a fixed prescription for action. The former chief executive of British Petroleum Tony Hayward would agree from his experience with BP's oil drilling disaster in the Gulf of Mexico. He could not have followed Johnson and Johnson in recalling spilled oil. But it did help him, albeit not decisively, to come clean and admit responsibility early in the saga, something that the management of Toyota failed to do. In sum, there are broad hidden rules in cases, but this does not reduce a case to a rigid set of rules, nor does it bind the decision-maker in each situation to follow all the rules.

7.3.1.2 *Case-based reasoning in medicine*

The applicability of case-based reasoning to medical diagnosis and choice of therapy seems obvious. The experienced medical practitioner, whether in the East or West, builds his competence on having compiled a library of cases in his own memory bank to which he can turn to almost intuitively as a habit of reasoning.

To charge these cases with the *post hoc ergo propter hoc* fallacy would seem to be too dismissive. Does it mean that experience gained from treating patients and observing experienced physicians treat their patients is of no help in improving a doctor's medical judgment, unless that experience is validated by controlled trials? This would fly in the face of common sense. This *reductio ad absurdum* argument however attacks a straw man. The experienced physician would have seen cases in which the same or similar treatments were not given and noted the negative outcomes. In effect, each past case seen by the physician (or by others whose reports he has read) is a member of a sample for implicit observational trials. Hence the value of cases is in providing samples of patients that receive a given treatment compared to those who did not.

Cases, therefore, when properly recorded and analysed, potentially contain data for the methods (other than RCTs) of evidence-based medicine.

In Chinese medicine, case studies have historically been an important form of transmitting knowledge in medicine as they contain a wealth of medical records. In China, such studies date back to the Han dynasty and in Greek medicine even earlier to Hippocrates *(Epidemics)*. In the 16th century, physicians in China started to write medical cases in a formal disciplined format, detailing the symptoms of the patient and the physician's diagnosis, and the rationale for the prescribed treatments.[198] Can one find valid evidence for TCM theory in the tens of thousands of classical case studies recorded by famous physicians from ancient times, for example by extracting data to form observational trials?

It would be difficult for these classical case studies in TCM to be sources of evidence for TCM methods. For a start, there have been lurking suspicions, even among TCM physicians. Why are nearly all the cases those of successful treatments and how many cases of failure have not been recorded? Were the putative cures permanent, or were there relapses among patients who sought treatment from other physicians, or whose illnesses progressed and eventually killed them? Were they mainly guilty of the *post hoc ergo propter hoc* fallacy? Because the patient got better following the application of a particular treatment method, we add it to the database of successful cases, precisely the kind of fallacious reasoning that RCTs are designed to avoid. Finally, there is the unhappy history of therapies like blood-letting that were thought in the past to have been validated through case studies for a variety of illnesses and later turned out on more rigorous examination to be useless in nearly all of them.

7.3.2 *Observational studies in Chinese medicine*

The situation is different, however, for recorded cases of modern Chinese physicians working in clinics where data is available on

---

[198] See, for example, Cullen (2001:309–321).

the progress of each patient through a complete course of treatment, sometimes lasting several years of treatment, until the patient has fully recovered or has moved on.[199] With more reliable data now available from large numbers of patients at state-run TCM hospitals and clinics in China and with TCM physicians assisted by technical staff and obliged to keep detailed and accurate records, there is potential for rigorous observational studies with adequate sample sizes to be conducted. The data studied must of course include contrast classes within which a medical intervention under study is not applied.

In principle, observational studies based on medical cases are possible using statistical and data mining techniques of the social sciences.[200] As a simple example of statistical analysis of case data, one can test the hypothesis that the herb *huangqin* (*radix scutellariae*) clears internal heat in the lungs. A random sample is created from past cases in which *huangqin* was used as part of various formulations for treating patients with internal heat in the lungs. A suitable method of statistical analysis would then be used. For example, multiple regression analysis could be used to determine the statistical significance of the *huangqin* factor in reducing lung heat. The regression methodology implicitly builds in a contrast class into the study. If *huangqin* emerges as a statistically significant variable, this would lend support to the proposition that using *huangqin* is more likely to achieve a heat reduction outcome than if it is not.

It is to be hoped that more research resources will be put into such studies. As for ancient case records of famous physicians, it

---

[199] See, for example, cardiovascular disease cases treated with Chinese medicine in Becker *et al.* (2005).

[200] Data mining is the process of applying computer science methods such as neural networks, cluster analysis and decision trees to data with the intention of uncovering hidden pattern in large data sets.

is likely that these cases will be taken on faith by TCM physicians and employed as tools for training new physicians rather than a valid source of evidence for TCM theory.

7.4 Evidence from TCM: Summing up

TCM models of therapy based on syndrome differentiation constitute the core theory of TCM; these models can and should be put to the test through clinical trials if TCM is to be considered a scientific system of healing. Clinical trials can be done in a variety of ways and need not be limited to RCTs.

To be sure are some methodological difficulties in using double-blind RCTs to test TCM interventions, but they do not amount to a need to reject them for testing TCM. Rather they should be used selectively, as should observational trials. Classical case studies of famous physicians are useful as pedagogical tools for training TCM physicians, but they do not provide a reliable database for observational trials. Properly-kept detailed records of modern TCM clinics and hospitals with large patient bases are more promising for this purpose.

Chapter 8

Placebo Effects and Cultural Factors

One of the most successful physicians I have ever known has assured me
that he used more bread pills, drops of coloured water, and powders
of hickoryashes, than of all other medicines put together.

Thomas Jefferson

Placebo effects exist in TCM as they do in Western interventions. RCTs aim, among other things, to determine if the effects of interventions are significantly higher than those of placebos.

This chapter discusses the placebo effect in TCM and how cultural factors might play a role in patient response to TCM interventions. The arguments and observations made here do not directly impinge on the core theme of the last chapter, which advocated conducting clinical trials on TCM models of therapy as the means of establishing the scientific validity (or otherwise) of these models. Instead they aim to elucidate a cultural aspect of TCM that makes the placebo effect possibly stronger than Western intervention in many conditions.

8.1 Discovery of Placebo Effects

Although placebos in the past were originally defined by their presumed inert content and their use as controls in clinical trials, recent research suggests that placebo effects are real physiological events occurring within a therapeutic context. Placebo effects can

187

also exist in clinical conditions even if no placebo is administered.[201]

There is an extensive literature on placebo effects found in clinical trials and on the theoretical mechanism of action of the placebo. Before the Second World War, the term 'placebo' referred to the harmless (sugar or bread) pills and tonics that doctors sometimes used to humour patients who had no obvious illness but still requested treatment. This practice was justified on the grounds that it did no harm even if it did nothing physically to help the patient get better. After the war, and with the rise to prominence of the double-blind RCTs, there was increasing recognition that the placebo could have powerful therapeutic effects at least in some circumstances and for some conditions. Beecher in fact claimed that placebos could induce "gross physical change", including changes which "may exceed those attributable to potent pharmacological action".[202] Kaptchuk dramatizes this point as a change of the status of the placebo from the "humble humbug" to potent stuff with occult-like powers that could mimic potent drugs.[203]

The thesis of placebos having real therapeutic effects was challenged by a number of studies, one of which pointed out a methodological flaw in Beecher's paper: nearly all his cases compared a prescribed treatment with a placebo and did not include a group with no treatment, leaving open the possibility that the observed supposed placebo effect was merely a result of the natural progression of the disease, that is, it would have happened even without the placebo. Hrobjartsson and Gotzsche subsequently conducted a meta-analysis of 130 clinical trials involving both a

---

[201] Finniss *et al.* (2010).
[202] Beecher (1955).
[203] Kaptchuk (1998).

placebo group and a no-treatment group. Because a sufficiently large number of conditions studies did not respond to the placebo, they concluded that there was no statistically significant evidence that placebos have clinical therapeutic effects.[204] But as Dylan Evans points out, all that the authors succeeded in showing was that the placebo is not a panacea that works for every conceivable condition or even a majority of conditions. (For that matter, no conventional drug claims to be a panacea for all ills.)[205]

To establish the placebo effect, one only has to single out the pathological conditions for which a placebo would make a significant difference. Thus, although Beecher's stronger claim that the placebo can affect every medical condition was not borne out by evidence from later studies, this left open the possibility that there are a range of conditions that are placebo-responsive. In fact, in the Hrobjartsson and Gotzsche study, pain was a condition that quite consistently responded positively to a placebo. This point is worth noting when we consider acupuncture for the treatment of pain, undoubtedly the most common application of acupuncture procedures. For certain conditions, such as anxiety, the results were variable and did not permit a firm interpretation. Thus, meta-analyses involving the pooling of results of studies of a variety of medical conditions tend to obscure the true profile of the placebo response.

Placebo mechanisms can interact with active treatments since every treatment is given in a therapeutic context that may activate placebo mechanisms working through similar biochemical pathways to those of the actual drug. Finniss *et al.* report an experimental trial done on post-operative pain during which patients were given intravenous saline as placebo in addition to

---

[204] In Kienle and Kiene (1997).
[205] Evans (2005).

routine analgesic treatment. One group was told that the infusion was merely a rehydrating solution and another group told that it was a strong painkiller. The group who believed the solution was assisting in analgesia took 33% less analgesic for the same pain control than did those in the control group, suggesting a clinical placebo effect working in conjunction with an active treatment to reduce the patient's overall drug intake.[206]

Various explanations have been offered for the action mechanism of a placebo. Evans has offered the controversial thesis that the placebo response involves the suppression of "the acute-phase response". This refers to the classic signs of inflammation (swelling, heat, redness and pain) together with the psychological symptoms of sickness behaviour (lethargy, apathy, loss of appetite and increased sensitivity to pain). Evans argues that this explanation is backed by his observation that the most frequently encountered placebo-responsive conditions are pain, swelling, stomach ulcers, depression and anxiety.[207] Finniss, *et al.* (2010) list a dozen or so mechanisms that could be involved in the placebo effect, ranging from the release of endogenous opioids and dopamine for pain reduction to the conditioning of immune system mediators like lymphocytes. For a given medical condition, one or more, or all, of these mechanisms could be at play. For each situation in which there is a placebo effect at play, a certain number of these mechanisms are sufficient to bring about therapeutic effect. In terms of the INUS concept and causal pie model (Chapter 2), we can view the placebo effect to be the result of the ability of the mind to trigger a certain constellation of psychobiological mechanisms, each of which is an 'insufficient but non-redundant part of an unnecessary but sufficient (INUS) condition' for a healing effect.

---

[206] Finniss *et al.* (2010).
[207] Evans (2003:44–69).

8.2 Placebo Effect in TCM

The placebo effect in alternative medicine in general, and in TCM in particular, has been the subject of considerable empirical research.[208] Studies involving placebo-controlled trials vary widely in methodological rigour and comprehensiveness. Many claim to have detected placebo effects, and a large number suggest that the placebo effect might be the *only* one that is significant. A study by Shang *et al.* of 136 placebo-controlled clinical trials concludes that "the effectiveness of Chinese herbal medicine remains poorly documented."[209]

Kaptchuk observes that Western medical scientists often suspect that the effectiveness of Chinese medicine is due to the placebo effect but contends that in China it is Western medicine that has the prestige and "an aura of the mysterious and foreign" and therefore may enjoy an advantage when it comes to inducing a placebo response.[210] I think the cultural factor cuts both ways depending on the illness and the kind of patient involved. Among the Chinese who believe in TCM, a majority of whom have had schooling in modern science, there is the perception that Western medicine is powerful and fast-acting, often with toxic side effects, eliminating symptoms but not the underlying (root) cause. Unless the body is able to readjust its balance internally and overcome the underlying cause, the illness is likely to return. Examples of such conditions would be the chronic headache which an analgesic like paracetamol can relieve but only for a couple of hours, and gastric pain relieved by an antacid that returns once gastric secretion levels rise again. TCM believers view TCM treatments

---

[208] See a survey by Shang *et al.* (2007: 1086) of some of the recent findings and Wu (2010).

[209] Shang (2007:1086).

[210] Kaptchuk (2000:33, footnote 27).

as attacking the root of the problem, taking longer but bringing about a more permanent cure. For example, TCM theory attributes headaches to a variety of underlying syndromes, among which are deficiency of *qi*, causing inadequate nourishment to the head, and liver heat which rises to the head to cause pain. TCM treatment would provide a *qi* tonic for the first case, and dissipate heat in the second; in each case it would claim to be removing the source of the pain rather than suppressing the pain.

For TCM patients, it could thus be argued that the placebo effect is stronger with Western medicine for short-term relief of acute conditions but not so for chronic illnesses. This might well be an explanation for conventional wisdom among TCM users that one should go to a Western doctor for an acute illness and to TCM physician for chronic conditions. If indeed the placebo effect was stronger in TCM interventions for chronic illnesses among believers, it does not of course rule out the existence of real therapeutic effects as well. Alongside strong placebo effects, such real effects would further influence TCM believers towards TCM interventions for chronic illnesses.

There may be other reasons for thinking that the role of the placebo effect may be stronger for TCM than it is for Western medicine. For one, patients who have not obtained satisfactory results from Western therapy often seek alternative therapy with the hope (and desire to believe) that it would work for them. For example, many TCM patients suffering from neck, shoulder and back pains do not recover by using anti-inflammatory drugs, or are unable to tolerate the side effects of these drugs (usually on their digestive systems); or they do not find relief in conventional physiotherapy. They seek the help of alternative medicine after hearing favourable anecdotal reports from others. These patients tend to cling to the hope and come with a higher level of optimism that acupuncture and related alternative therapies would give them the relief that has eluded them with conventional therapy. Take as an example the influenza patient mentioned in Chapter 1 who recovers after treatment by a Western doctor with an antipyretic for fever and antibiotics for secondary bacterial infection but suffers post-flu chronic dry cough and lassitude. He believes that the TCM would fix his problem. The TCM physician treats his dry cough as a deficiency syndrome in the lung-*yin* and lassitude as arising from damaged *qi*. If he recovers quickly, he might be inclined to regard this as a vindication of TCM for chronic conditions.

Another reason is that alternative therapists tend to spend more time with their patients than do conventional doctors (40 minutes versus 17 minutes); they also engage in more direct physical contact than doctors who prescribe pills after a quick examination.[211] The higher perceived level of empathy for their patients is likely to evoke a stronger placebo response.

Third, in Eastern cultures, TCM patients tend not only to be strong believers in TCM therapy, but can also relate better to the terms and language used by Chinese physicians without the problems of translation of these terms that a non-Chinese speaker would experience. This is particularly so with respect to the differentiation of TCM syndromes and their treatment. The average Chinese patient in China or Singapore, for example, has little problem understanding the physicians who tell him that he suffers from *qi* deficiency or damp heat, but may have more difficulty understanding blood test results that show a low platelet count or an elevated ESR. Explanations offered by the TCM physician to the patient of the underlying problem of his illness and the method adopted to tackle it builds confidence of the patient in the physician and may well evoke a stronger placebo response.

---

[211] Evans (2003:157–158).

If indeed it is true that the placebo effect on average is much stronger with TCM treatments than Western medical treatments, then the true therapeutic effect of the TCM treatment would be harder to tease out from clinical trials because of the swamping effect of the placebo response and because the two effects may not be linearly additive. For example, suppose on a scale of 10 to 1 the placebo effect acting alone reduces the pain level from 10 to 5. Suppose further that the prescribed TCM treatment acting alone reduces it from 10 to 7. The combined effect of placebo and treatment would not necessarily reduce pain level from 10 to 2, perhaps only from 10 to 4. (By analogy, two teaspoonful of sugar would not necessarily make your tea *taste* twice as sweet as one teaspoonful, and for people who do not like sugar in their tea one teaspoonful might taste just as awful; nor would a punch of the face with half the force of a boxer's fist be felt as only half as painful as one received with full force.) In the above example, the additional 1 point reduction from TCM treatment would be that much harder to isolate by statistical inference.

One can only speculate whether or not the foregoing observation is an explanation for a plethora of Western studies pointing to pain as among the conditions most placebo-responsive to Chinese acupuncture. For example, a series of large trials in Germany compared Chinese medical acupuncture, sham acupuncture (needling at non-acupuncture points) and no treatment for conditions varying from migraine and tension headaches to chronic low back pain and osteoarthritis of the knee.[212] Generally across the various trials, outcomes did not differ between Chinese and sham acupuncture groups although both of these fared better than the no-treatment group. In four of these RCTs, the patient's

---

[212] Linde *et al.* (2005), Melchart D, Streng A, Hoppe A, *et al.* (2005), Brinkhaus B, Witt CM, Jena S, *et al.* (2006), Haake *et al.* (2007).

expectation of pain relief was the best predictor of efficacy of treatment, irrespective of whether genuine Chinese or sham acupuncture was applied.[213]

In contrast, most studies in China and East Asia (notably Hong Kong, Macao, Taiwan and South Korea) suggest that there was more than a placebo effect at play with genuine Chinese acupuncture. Such studies are regularly reported in Chinese journals like the *Chinese Journal of Integrative Medicine, American Journal of Chinese Medicine,* and dozens of official journals of TCM colleges and universities in the country. These "uniformly favourable" trial result have raised doubts over the reliability of scientific evidence from these studies.[214]

While no one is likely to deny that pain is placebo-responsive to acupuncture, more work remains to be done using common accepted clinical trial protocols before clear conclusions can be drawn regarding the existence of significant non-placebo effects of acupuncture.

---

[213] Linde *et al.* (2007).

[214] Kaptchuk (2000: Appendix E, 357).

Chapter 9

Conclusion: TCM Theory Reinterpreted

The aim of philosophy is to show the fly out of the fly-bottle.
Ludwig Wittgentstein

Chinese medical theory has been under attack since the May 4th movement of 1919 in China, first by Chinese youth newly armed with Western science and technology, and later by scientists in the West influenced by the philosophical positivism of the Vienna Circle and of Karl Popper. It enjoyed a brief respite after Chairman Mao decreed it as 'a treasure trove of Chinese wisdom' and ordered its modernisation, taking into account advances in Western medicine and, where possible, integrating it with the latter. But as colleges of TCM flourished in China and spread to other East Asian countries as well as to the West, challenges to its scientific credentials grew more strident from a generation of biomedical scientists nurtured on the reductionism of molecular and cellular biology and vaunting the statistical power of the new evidence-based medicine.

Part of the problem faced by Western medical scientists in understanding TCM has been the terminology used, which is not helped by the difficulties in translation. But the main difficulty is the lack of understanding of the underlying meanings of TCM concepts and entities, which tend to become ambiguous and

197

suspiciously metaphysical when attempts are made to define them in observable and measurable terms.

The other major problem has been the paucity of evidence that Chinese therapeutic methods actually work — evidence that would be acceptable by the standards and methods of evidence-based medicine. The problem has been exacerbated by some defenders of TCM theory who try to avoid the rigours of evidence-based medicine with the excuse that TCM theory is a different 'paradigm' from Western medicine and therefore absolved from the latter's rules of evidence.

This book has tried to show how TCM theory may be reconstructed to make sense to biomedical science and to assess the evidential credentials of the thus reconstructed theory, in particular, to see if the efficacy of the therapeutic methods derived from the theory can be put to scientific testing through clinical trials.

On the nature of TCM entities, we saw in Chapters 4 and 5 that one does not need to be burdened by the thought of key entities like *qi*, phlegm and meridians being ambiguous and unobservable. Nor should one be disconcerted by that fact that a vital organ like the kidney in TCM is very different from the kidney in modern anatomy. TCM entities should be treated as comprising real substances, like blood and bone, and also as theoretical constructs or abstractions of real underlying biomedical substances and processes, like *jing* and *qi*. TCM organs are systems of functions rather than the somatic structures of modern anatomy. These abstractions and theoretical constructs evolved over the long history of Chinese medical theory and practice. They constitute building blocks for TCM models that are used for explaining, diagnosing and treating of illnesses.

To speak of these abstractions as if they were real observable entities accounts for the conceptual distress encountered by new

Western readers of Chinese medical literature. On the other hand, terms like 'analogies', 'metaphors' and van Frassen-inspired empirically adequate "convenient fictions" used on TCM entities may be helpful for inducting the lay reader into TCM thought.[215] But when used as general characterisations of TCM entities they are often inaccurate and in some instances misleading.

The problem is further compounded by the habit in Chinese culture of using language in more flexible ways than is encountered in English grammar, coupled with a tendency to blur distinctions between substance, energy and process. This has led to imaginative ways to explain TCM concepts, like treating them as poetic images, an approach that indeed can be helpful but only for the new reader to get acquainted with TCM without the need for 'epistemological leaps' from his conceptual base in biomedicine.

TCM theory is expressed through models that attempt to elucidate what a healthy state of the body consists of. It offers its own explanations of the causes of illness and provides a system for diagnosis and treatment of illnesses. Although some TCM models evolved from ancient cosmology and folklore, this does not change the fact that, as used today, they are heuristic models based on empirical observations in clinical practice. As heuristic models, they are conjectures about what governs events in the human body viewed somewhat like the black box in cybernetics. These events manifest themselves through constellations of clinical symptoms that TCM physicians differentiate as patterns or *syndromes*. These syndromes are then treated with therapeutic principles for resolving the syndromes, applied using a variety of natural products (including herbs, minerals and animal parts), acupuncture interventions and medical massage (*tuina*).

---

[215] van Frassen (1980).

The case for the usefulness and scientific credibility of TCM models must rest on the usefulness of these models in diagnosis and treatment tested through clinical trials. Because of the complexity of the human body and TCM's dependence on human observation rather than objective blood tests and diagnostic instruments, and because of the dynamic nature of TCM syndromes, there are challenging though not insurmountable methodological problems in running clinical trials on TCM models. The problems are compounded by TCM being patient-centric, hence heavily biased toward individualised treatment. There is also a possibly stronger placebo effect for TCM therapies than conventional ones, making the real impact of the treatment harder to tease out and isolate from their joint effect.

There is a good case for making more use of observational trials for testing TCM therapy models. Insisting on employing only double-blind randomised controlled trials (RCTs) is to ignore the limited feasibility of such trials in practice and to place RCTs on an unwarranted high pedestal relative to other kinds of clinical trials.

Clinical trials on TCM methods are still in their infancy despite considerable efforts in both Western and Eastern research institutions. This is largely because nearly all of this work has been directed at what should rightly be termed 'Western herbal treatments' and 'Western acupuncture' rather than being focused on TCM models based on syndrome differentiation. This leaves much more clinical work to be done to directly address TCM theory. It calls for investigations into whether TCM models are at least approximately valid under specified constraints.

The current lack of rigorously collected evidence for the efficacy of interventions based on TCM theory places it a notch below economic science in the scientific hierarchy. Despite the presence of contending theories, the frequent failed model, and doubts over the feasibility of modelling complex economic and social activity encountered in economic science, 'the dismal science' has earned a measure of credibility through statistical testing of its models and occasional successes of these models in prediction.

It is hard to agree with orthodox thinkers in Chinese medicine who treat ancient classics as special infallible insights into the working of the human body attained through introspection and more than a hint of divine inspiration. Although it is helpful to see Chinese medicine as having some paradigms (exemplars in the sense of the later Kuhn) that are different from those of Western medicine, there is little value in pressing the stronger claim that Chinese medicine itself is a different paradigm from, and incommensurable with, that of Western medicine. Nor is there any justification for the view that because some TCM entities are unobservable or have escaped scientific observation they are therefore absolved from the rigours of evidence-based medicine.

My reconstruction of TCM theory recognises the ontological status of TCM entities as a mixed bag of real biomedical entities and theoretical abstractions of these entities, but with all of them ultimately derived from real physiological functions and activities. The heuristic models used in TCM need to be validated by success in clinical practice and confirmed through appropriate clinical trials. They have to be tested and refined. Some of them, including the five-element model, may eventually be abandoned. What should emerge is a set of constructions and empirical models that together constitute a holistic non-reductionist way of organising observations of body functioning and pathology to serve as tools for diagnosis and therapy.

Whether these tools can be shown through scientific evidence to be of significant value towards cultivating good health and curing illnesses remains to be seen. Should some of them be proven valuable to the satisfaction of modern scientists — and I would venture to say that it is unlikely that of none of them be proven to be of value — it is probable to be for promoting a more holistic and a patient-centric approach to health cultivation and the management of chronic illnesses.

Chapter 10

TCM Treatment of Chronic Illnesses

*The good physician treats the disease; the great physician treats
the patient who has the disease.*

William Osler

TCM is extensively used in East Asian countries, and to some
extent in Australia, Europe and North America, as complementary
treatment for certain chronic illnesses. In less acute cases, it is
often also used as an alternative to Western treatments.

To illustrate how TCM methods are applied to some common chronic illnesses, we examine briefly below its use in coronary heart disease, strokes, digestive disorders and irritable bowel
syndrome, as well as depression. These conditions have been
chosen because TCM treatment in each case provides an interesting complement or alternative, or a combination of both, to
Western medicine. TCM physicians regularly encounter patients
who may not have found satisfactory results with Western medicine for such ailments and seek complementary or alternative
treatments.

The objective here is not to demonstrate the viability of TCM
methods — this would in any case require difficult and complex
clinical trials — but rather to show how TCM methods have been
used in a wide variety of clinical work and, where possible, offer

a biomedical interpretation of why these methods might conceivably have brought relief to patients.

10.1 Coronary Heart Disease

In most instances coronary heart disease involves the narrowing of blood vessels supplying nutrients and oxygen to the heart, this narrowing is caused by dietary, genetic, ageing and lifestyle factors with build-up of fatty plaque on arterial walls. Angina pain can occur when blood supply is inadequate and cardiac arrest when there is constriction or blockage.

TCM interprets coronary heart disease as an impediment or blockage of the free flow of *qi* and blood. The condition is classified under 'chest blockage with heart pain' (*xiongbi xintong* 胸痹 心痛) in TCM textbooks and attributed to one or more of seven underlying syndromes, of which the most common are deficiency of heart-*qi* and blood stasis.[216]

The syndrome of 'deficiency of heart-*qi*' is identified by symptoms of dull pain in the chest, heart palpitations, shortness of breath which worsens upon exertion, fatigue and sweating without exertion; the tongue is pale and slightly swollen, with tooth indentations and thin white fur; the pulse is slow, weak and thready or slow and irregular. The syndrome of 'blood stasis' has symptoms of stabbing pain or angina pains in the chest, sometimes spreading to the back and shoulders; it can be accompanied by prolonged chest oppression; the tongue is dark with ecchymosis (bluish-black marks) and thin fur; pulse is wiry and astringent, or rapid and intermittent/irregular. The first syndrome of deficient

---

[216] In Chinese, the syndromes are 心气不足, and 瘀血痹阻, 心阴亏顺, 痰浊闭阻. See, for example, a detailed description of TCM treatments for heart disease may be found in Becker *et al.* (2005).

heart-*qi* is consistent with early or mild coronary heart disease. Blood stasis syndrome is usually found in more advanced stages of the disease when significant atherosclerosis has set in.

Accordingly, TCM treatment for the first syndrome consists of strengthening the body's *qi* level and promoting (regulating) its flow through *qigong* and *taiji* exercises, as well as diets containing foods and herbs that tonify *qi*, such as American ginseng (*xiyangshen* 西洋参), wild yam (*huaishan* 淮山) Astragalus (*huangqi* 黄芪), *Panax Ginsena* (renshen 人参), *Radix Condonopsis* (*dangshen* 党参) and *Radix Notogingseng* (*sanqi* 三七). A typical prescription formulation, appropriately modified to suit each patient's condition, would be *Baoyuan Tang* 保元汤 combined with *Ganmaidazao Tang* 甘麦大枣汤. The first uses ginseng and Astragalus as the main components for boosting *qi* levels. The latter uses *Fructus Tritici Aestivi* (*xiaomai* 小麦 or wheat) as the monarch herb to nourish heart-*yin* and roasted liquorice (*zhigancao* 炙甘草) as the minister herb to promote flow along the heart meridian, invigorating the heart and tranquilising the mind.[217]

For the second syndrome, TCM treatment would typically encourage the consumption of foods and herbs that improve blood circulation and reduce blood stasis. These would include *Radix Salviae Miltiorrhizae* (*danshen* 丹参), hawthorn berries (*shanzha* 山楂), red yeast rice (*hongqumi* 红曲米), *Rhizoma Chuanxiong* (*chuanxiong* 川芎), *Flos Catharmi* (*honghua* 红花), *Semen Persicae* (*taoren* 桃仁), black fungus vegetable, turmeric and pomegranate fruit.[218] In biomedical terms, these herbs are

---

[217]The "monarch" herb in the main one and the "minister" herbs play the chief supporting function. See Chapter 11.

[218]Noted advocate of natural healing, Andrew Weil (M.D.) recommends the regular consumption of black fungus for coronary heart health. See Weil (1995:166).

known to have mild vasodilating effects, rendering transient improved blood flow and symptomatic relief from angina pains. In the TCM framework, such vasodilating effects are part of more lasting changes by 'resolving blood stasis', a claim which implies slower build-up of plaque and less impediment to blood flow.

A typical prescription for blood stasis syndrome in the chest is the 'Decoction for Removing Blood Stasis in the Chest' (*Xuefu Zhuyu Tang* 血府逐瘀汤). This formulation contains 11 herbs, with *honghua* and *taoren* as monarch drugs, and *chuanxiong* as one of the minister drugs. In recent years the classical Chinese formulation 'Danshen Dripping Pills" (*Fufang Danshen Diwan* 复方丹参滴丸) for alleviating blood stasis and improving blood flow has been subjected to FDA trials and is awaiting final approval for use in the treatment of coronary heart disease. This formulation contains *danshen, sanqi* and *Borneolum Syntheticum* (*bingpian* 冰片).

10.1.1 *Interpretation*

Compared to Western treatments using the nitrates for vasodilation, blood thinners (like aspirin) to reduce the risk of blood clots, and surgical interventions like angioplasty and bypass surgery, TCM treatments are slower and cannot deal effectively with acute angina or emergency situations of coronary infarction. But they could be useful either as complementary treatment or as an alternative to surgical intervention.

TCM treatments, with proper medical advice recognising drug contraindications and the condition of the patient, can and are being administered alongside Western treatments. TCM approaches to management of heart conditions using medicated diets and Chinese exercises can complement Western methods such as maintaining low cholesterol levels, exercises for cardiovascular fitness, and a diet rich in fibre and low in saturated and trans fats, with emphasis on fresh fruits and vegetables to promote endothelial health.

A biomedical explanation of the usefulness of TCM therapies for coronary heart disease would point to the possible effect of herbs and Chinese exercises on improving blood circulation and inhibiting atherosclerosis. In the practice of biomedicine, a school of cardiologists, sometimes referred to as 'integrated cardiologists', are doing pioneering work in using diet and dietary supplements that go beyond conventional tools of cholesterol reduction, blood-thinning, vasodilation with drugs, and surgical intervention to prevent cardiac events and enhance cardiac health. Some cardiologists advocate a de-emphasis of cholesterol reduction and point to other equally or more important risk factors like excessive lipoprotein(a) and homocystein and low levels of CoQ10. Others focus on food, particularly a vegetarian and low-oil diet. Research on TCM herbs point to a possible connection between herbs used for coronary heart disease and the improvement of endothelial health and reduction of inflammation that are critical to prevention and therapy for coronary heart disease.[219]

10.2 Hypertension and Stroke

With ageing, atherosclerosis sets in as arteries narrow with fatty plaque on their walls. The likelihood of suffering a stroke rises almost exponentially after the age of 65. Both Western medicine and TCM treat patients to prevent strokes and, if a stroke has occurred, to ameliorate its effects and improve quality of life. The

---

[219] See, for example, Sinatra and Roberts (2007), Campbell and Campbell (2004), and Esselstyn (2008). On yellow ginger or turmeric (curcumin) for heart health, see, for example, Akazawa *et al.* (2012) and Sinatra (2012).

approaches taken by the two systems of medicine appear radically different, but in fact have underlying commonalities.

Of the two major kinds of strokes, the ischaemic stroke and the haemorrhagic stroke, the former is by far the more common, being precipitated by sudden impeded blood flow in an artery of the brain. This could be caused by clotting at the artery (thrombosis), or a detached clot from another location — usually the heart or the carotid artery — that lodges itself within the artery (embolism), cutting off oxygen supply to part of the brain. A haemorrhagic stroke results from rupture of an artery wall, leading to cerebral haemorrhage, and it is commonly correlated with degenerative disease of the arteries and hypertension. The use of blood thinners like warfarin can also raise the risk of a haemorrhagic stroke.

Western medicine attributes strokes to a combination of risk factors, which may include hypertension, smoking, excessive cholesterol (LDL) levels, and diabetes. Heart arrhythmia in the form of atrial fibrillation can also produce clots that travel to the brain.

TCM views that the underlying conditions predisposing a person to strokes involve the endogenous wind (*feng*) pathogen; hence the Chinese term for stroke is *zhongfeng*, or "attack by wind". Endogenous wind may arise from one or more of several factors, which include (a) weakness of *yin* and blood giving rise to liver heat and wind; (b) overwork and strain stirring up liver wind; (c) inappropriate diet that creates warm phlegm in the spleen, generating endogenous wind; (d) emotional stress particularly anger triggering fire and the production of harmful wind.[220]

---

[220] These standard explanations may be found in textbooks like Zhou (2007:304–310).

A large number of TCM syndrome combinations are associated with strokes, depending on the nature of the stroke and the stage of progression, whether at the onset, in the immediate aftermath, or during the longer term debilitated phase of the patient. At the onset and immediate aftermath stage, hyperactivity of liver-*yang*, phlegm with wind, and stirring of liver wind (*ganfeng neidong* 肝风内动) are the common syndromes; at the later recovery stages, phlegm and blood stasis are often present, and the patient may suffer from severe *qi* deficiency and weakness of the liver and kidney. *Tianma Gouteng Yin* (天麻钩藤饮) with suitable variations to suit the patient is most often used in the early stages whilst tonics with ingredients added for resolving blood stasis such as *Buyang Huanwu Tang* (补阳还五汤) are administered in the recovery stages. Thus, treatment of these TCM syndromes associated with strokes follows the principle of customising therapy to the syndrome and the constitution of the patient.

Treatment usually combines herbal prescriptions, acupuncture and *tuina*, and is continually varied as the internal state of the patient changes and new syndromes are exhibited. TCM theory explains that acupuncture helps the rehabilitation process by enhancing flow of *qi* and blood in the body, leading to better recovery of motor skills and overall physical functioning by inducing beneficial changes in the blood flow to the brain. Common points used in post-stroke acupuncture treatment include *taichong* 太冲, *hegu* 合谷, *renzhong* 人中, *baihui* 百会, *sanyinjiao* 三阴交, neiguan 内关, *yanglingquan* 阳陵泉 and *quchi* 曲池. These acupoints can also be used in the treatment of hypertension.

Exercises like *qigong* and *taijiquan*, for patients with sufficient mobility, are believed to enhance recovery from post-stroke disabilities. Social interaction within *qigong* groups may also help to improve patient morale and nurture the positive emotions that facilitate recovery.

10.2.1 *Interpretation*

Western medical explanations for stroke revolve around vascular impediments to blood flow and the contribution of diet, lifestyle and hypertension to precipitating cerebral thrombosis or embolism. TCM explanations centre on the TCM *gan* (liver) where endogenous wind may form as a result of deficiencies and imbalances in the body. These differing explanations are not necessarily incompatible; instead they represent alternative models for prevention and therapy.

Hypertension has a central role as the dominant risk factor in Western medical explanations for stroke. The causes of hypertension are complex: risk factors like diabetes, high dietary salt intake and emotional stress are well established but many cases of hypertension are idiopathic and a significant percentage of patients with the condition do not respond to drug treatment. The TCM syndrome of hyperactivity of liver-*yang*, which can lead to endogenous wind, has some resemblance to hypertension although wider in scope. It can be brought about by stress and emotional factors, but also by blood, *yin* and/or *qi* deficiencies, and the presence of phlegm. In this respect, TCM theory presents a wider menu of preventive measures for stroke that revolve around diet, emotional management, exercises to improve *qi* and blood levels/flows. TCM diagnosis of syndromes and body constitutions that predispose a person to stroke could possibly make the claim to offering a comprehensive prevention regimen by prescribing therapies to resolve or mitigate these syndromes.

A similar scenario prevails in the treatment of strokes. Western treatments rely heavily on blood coagulants like warfarin to prevent recurrence and on physiotherapy for rehabilitation. Chinese treatments directly address the prevailing syndromes at each stage of the evolution of the illness. In the early aftermath of a stroke, there is an emphasis on calming endogenous wind, in the later stages, the focus is on resolving phlegm and blood stasis, while in the rehabilitation and recovery phase, this shifts to tonics for *qi*, blood and the *yin* of the liver and kidney. Chinese exercises work on improving blood and *qi* circulation, postural robustness and joint mobility, less on building muscular strength. It would appear that a combination of Western and Chinese treatments would secure better results for the patient than a strict adherence to one regimen. When treatments are combined, there must be appropriate cognisance of drug compatibility, for example, the fact that some Chinese herbs have mild anticoagulant properties that may excessively enhance the effect of Western anticoagulant drugs.

10.3 Digestive Disorders and the Irritable Bowel Syndrome

Li Dongyuan（李东垣）of the *Jin-Yuan* dynasties focused on care of the digestive system for health and longevity. In TCM theory, digestion is largely captured by the *pi* (脾) organ, translated as the 'spleen'. However, the *pi* in TCM has little in common with the spleen of modern physiology. The TCM spleen governs the processing and transforming food into nutrients that feed other organs and the rest of the body, pairing with the *wei* 胃 (stomach) in its work. Damage to the spleen and stomach, in Li Dongyuan's framework, is the root cause of most illnesses.

The spleen in TCM nourishes the body and replenishes the store of *qi* and essence or *jing* in the vital organs. Growth and development in TCM theory are governed mainly by the *shen*

肾 (kidney). By providing nutrients to the *shen* to replenish the store of *qi* and *jing*, the *pi* serves as the foundation of post-natal health (*houtianzhiben* 后天之本). In addition, because of its direct supporting function for the lung as laid out in the five-element model, treating the spleen in clinical practice is sometimes the preferred route for the treatment of lung disorders. For example, chronic cough due to weak lung-*qi*, accompanied by white phlegm, poor appetite and fatigue, can be treated with spleen tonics. This nexus between the digestive system and the lung is important in TCM medical practice as chronic lung conditions would be deemed to be difficult to treat unless the digestive system (*pi*) was kept in good functioning order.

Adequate *qi* and its smooth flow are vital to the normal functions of the spleen. In TCM theory, spleen functions are inhibited by dampness, which is characterised by 'stickiness' that impedes the flow of *qi*, resulting in *qi* stagnation in the abdomen. With weak *qi* and/or *qi* stagnation, dampness accumulates further, food is not properly digested, and there could be resultant generation and accumulation of phlegm. Improper diet such as oily and fried foods and brooding accompanied by anxiety are the leading factors that damage the spleen, resulting in gastrointestinal disorders such as poor appetite, bloated abdomen, wind, loose stools, and the discomforts of the irritable bowel syndrome. The high incidence of digestive disorders in high-stress societies like New York, Beijing and Singapore may well be associated with stressful lifestyles that harm the spleen.

Herbal supplements used to strengthen spleen functions include dried tangerine peels (*chenpi* 陈皮), *sharen* (砂仁) and *banxia* (半夏) which are thought to smoothen the flow of spleen-*qi* and resolve dampness and phlegm; *dangshen* (党参), wild yam (*shanyao* 山药), *huangqi* (黄芪) and red dates (*dazao* 大枣) are used to tonify spleen-*qi*. These herbs can be used as food ingredients for spleen- healthy meals, although *sharen* and *banxia* are not so tasty and tend to be used more in medical prescriptions. A delicious and nourishing rice porridge with *huangqi*, red dates and wild yam is sometimes used to maintain healthy functioning of the spleen and stomach.

Common formulations for spleen disorders include *Sijunzi Tang, Shenling Baizhu San,* and *Xiangsha Liujunzi Tang.* [221] These formulations combine *qi* tonics with *qi* regulation and removal of dampness.

The Irritable Bowel Syndrome (IBS) is a recurrent condition with abdominal pains and constipation and/or diarrhoea, often with bloating of the abdomen and dyspepsia. There is no detectable structural disease. It can continue for years. The condition is often associated with stress or anxiety and may follow an episode of intestinal infection. From the point of view of Western medicine, "the cause is unknown".[222]

TCM regards IBS (*changyijizonghezheng* 肠易激综合征) as a condition associated with imbalances and/or stagnation in the spleen. It is not a disease in its own right, but one of several manifestations of imbalance and *qi* stagnation in the spleen. This could take the form of dampness in the spleen when spleen-*qi* is weak or does not flow properly, the result of improper diet or exposure to the dampness pathogen. It can also be the consequence of an 'exuberant' liver over-restraining the spleen (*ganwangchengpi*肝旺乘脾), a situation implied by the five-element model, causing the spleen to malfunction in its digestive role. The exuberant liver is often the result of stress and anxiety, causing stagnation in liver-*qi* flow and progressing to 'liver fire'. IBS is

---

[221] See Chapter 10 and Annex 2.
[222] Oxford Concise Medical Dictionary (2007:380).

frequently encountered in TCM practice especially among city dwellers in high-stress environments. Stress harms the liver, stoking exuberance and fire. Excessive consumption of fried and high-fat foods that are difficult to digest make a veritable breeding ground for spleen dampness.

TCM treatment for IBS comprises mainly resolving spleen dampness with herbs and formulations like *Xiangsha Liujunzi Tang,* or calming the liver with *Xiaoyaosan* with variations customised to the condition of the patient.[223] IBS-like conditions are frequently encountered in TCM clinical work and there is considerable anecdotal evidence of the efficacy of TCM treatments. Some clinical trials have claimed success with such treatments.[224]

10.3.1 *Interpretation*

If clinical trials indicate a high rate of success of TCM treatments for digestive disorders and IBS and related disorders, then biomedical explanations for the mechanisms of these treatment would present interesting research opportunities. TCM theory relates the action of certain herbs to syndromes of 'spleen dampness'. A biomedical interpretation would be that the constellation of symptoms differentiated as the spleen dampness syndrome was found from clinical experience to be relieved by certain herbs and formulations incorporating these herbs. These herbs were consequently classified as 'dampness resolving medications'. Without needing to invoke TCM theory, researchers would note from clinical experience and clinical trials that certain herbs are

---

[223] See Chapter 11 for a description of *Xiangsha Liujunzi Tang* and Annex 2 on *Xiaoyaosan.*
[224] For example, Bensoussan *et al.* (1998).

able to relieve symptoms associated with spleen dampness, including IBS. Such evidence would merely be seen as clinical findings that suggest the efficacy of certain herbs used as drugs for digestive disorders. Pharmacological research that reveals explanatory mechanisms for their therapeutic action would not directly conflict with TCM theory but should be seen as merely confirming the usefulness of the relevant TCM methods derived from TCM theory.

10.4 Depression

Depression in Western medicine is a mood disorder "characterised by the pervasive and persistent presence of core and somatic symptoms on most days for at least two weeks."[225] Core symptoms include impairment of motivation, energy and enjoyment, impaired memory, insomnia, loss of appetite and libido, and mood swings. A definitive diagnosis of clinical depression is difficult because symptoms vary greatly across individuals.

Western medicine views genetics, chronic illnesses and stress as possible underlying causes of depression. Depressive states may be accompanied by low levels of neurotransmitters in the parasympathetic nervous system. Treatment makes extensive use of anti-depressants, cognitive behavioural therapy and/or psychotherapy.

From the point of view of Chinese medicine, depression involves impediments to natural flows of blood and *qi* in the body; hence the key to overcoming depression is to restore healthy flows. The word *yu* 郁 means stagnation or the absence of smooth flow of *qi* in the body and the TCM term *yubing* 郁病 refers to a group of conditions arising from blocked flows in the

---

[225] Oxford Concise Medical Dictionary (2007:195).

body, leading to a variety of symptoms ranging from sadness and anxiety to vile tempers and autism. *Yubing* does not therefore correspond exactly to the Western medical meaning of depression and is best viewed as a class of syndromes, many of them exhibiting the symptoms associated with depression.

A common cause of *qi* stagnation in TCM theory is the emotional factor. Excessive anger and emotional stress leads to stagnation of liver-*qi*, which may progress into liver fire. Anxiety may result in the stagnation of spleen-*qi*, which in turn may encourage production of dampness and phlegm that further impede the flow of *qi*. Among menopausal and post-partum women who tend to be low in *yin* and *qi*, weakness or deficiency of blood and nourishment to the heart are commonly encountered. Depression-like symptoms include frequent abrupt mood swings, paranoia, anxiety and panic attacks.

The TCM approach to treatment of *yubing* involves identifying the blockages and imbalances and resolving them with herbal medications and/or acupuncture to restore *qi* flow. For mild cases, herbs with soothing and calming effects, targeting the particular syndrome exhibited by the patient, may be helpful. Herbs that help to improve *qi* flows include *Radix Bupleuri* (*chaihu* 柴胡), *Rhizoma Cyperi* (*xiangfu* 香附), *Citrus Medica* (*foshou* 佛手), *Cortex Albiziae* (*hehuanpi* 合欢皮) and *Rosa Rugosa* (*meiguihua* 玫瑰花). A simple recipe for calming with a drink of herbal tea uses rose and jasmine flowers, which have the actions of soothing the liver and dispersing *qi* stagnation of the liver, thereby alleviating symptoms such as chest tightness, tension and anxiety.

Common prescriptions used in treating depression include *Chaihushugansan* 柴胡疏肝散, *Xiaoyaosan* 逍遥散 for alleviating depression associated with blocked *qi* flows in the TCM 'liver' (*gan*) whereas *Ganmaidazao Tang* 甘麦大枣汤 is generally used in blood deficiency syndrome commonly seen in menopausal or post-partum women with frequent mood swings.

10.4.1 *Interpretation*

A biomedical interpretation of the claimed therapeutic effects of TCM treatments for depression may lie in the effects of these herbs in producing neurotransmitters and sustaining their levels in the parasympathetic nervous system. For example the seed of *Ziziphus Spinosa Hu* (*suanzaoren* 酸枣仁) has been found to be related to melatonin, a derivative of serotonin which is a key neurotransmitter for calming the body. Such explanations are likely to be incomplete, as the restoration of smooth *qi* flows in TCM implies a better functioning in general of physiological processes in the body — improved motility in digestion, enhanced sleep quality and a higher level of energy; these combine to produce a better feeling of well-being, encouraging the patient's own mind to overcome depressive moods.

10.5 Conclusion

In all the four cases above, TCM provides both complementary and alternative treatments to common chronic illnesses, working largely from the vantage point of restoring imbalances in the body system and encouraging the body's own healing powers to ameliorate the symptoms or bring about recovery. It is patient-centric in the sense of addressing directly the nature of the underlying syndromes present and adapting to changing syndromes as the illnesses evolve and progress in each patient.

Millions of patients around the world receive TCM treatments to relieve their sufferings and many more practise its system of health cultivation based on balance and natural flows in the body. Despite its ancient origins, TCM has shown remarkable resilience in preserving a healthcare role in modern scientific societies. This is unlikely to be attributable entirely to the power of superstition or the placebo effect. TCM treatments should be carefully and rigorously researched. Its more contentious claims should be scientifically and critically assessed and its efficacious aspects better understood and prudently applied.

Chapter 11

Chinese Medicinal Herbs

Drink one cupful of the [ginseng] mixture as a dose twice a day. Keep this up for 100 days. Then the person will have sharp eyesight and hearing, strong bones full of marrow, moistened and lustrous skin, and a powerful memory.

Bencao Gangmu

This chapter provides explanations of TCM herbal medications and theories guiding their use. Information on common herbs and formulations are provided in the annexes.

11.1 Chinese *Materia Medica* (Herbs)

Medicinal herbs have been used in Chinese medical practice for health promotion and treatment of illnesses for thousands of years. The properties and nature of these herbs and their therapeutic effects have been carefully studied and documented by over a hundred generations of herbalists and physicians. The earliest extant manual on herbs was written by the legendary Shen Nong of the Western Han dynasty (201 BC–AD 24) in the classic *Shennong Herbal Manual* (*Shennong Bencao Jing* 神农本草经). This contained detailed descriptions of 365 herbs which he came across in his travels over fields and mountains all over the country. Shen Nong personally tested these herbs on himself for toxicity and side effects at considerable risk to his life and health. During the Ming dynasty in 1578, the most comprehensive record of Chinese herbs to date was compiled, which has since then served as a reference text by Chinese physicians and pharmacists. *The Compendium of Materia Medica* (*Bencao Gangmu* 本草纲目) covered 1,892 herbs (inclusive of those of animal and mineral origins). The encyclopaedic nature of these scholarly works testifies to the empirical scientific tradition in Chinese medicine which relies on clinical evidence provided by detailed observation, record and analysis.

In modern times, most of these herbs have been analysed in the laboratory and in clinical trials for therapeutic properties, toxicity and side effects and the accumulation of these studies and the experience of earlier generations of physicians have been carefully documented in modern texts on Chinese medicinal herbs. Much work remains to be done as the variety of herbs is very large and their complexity of a much higher order of magnitude as a single herb typically contains dozens and sometimes over a hundred different ingredients and molecules in contrast to Western drugs that mainly comprise a single effective chemical (the 'active ingredient') for each drug.

11.1.1 *Classification of herbs*

Herbs can be classified according to their natural characteristics, or according to their therapeutic effects.

11.1.1.1 *Classification by natural characteristics*

The natural characteristics of herbs include their properties, flavours and meridian tropism (*guijing* 归经), the latter being an indication of the meridians along which the herb's therapeutic effects prefer to travel.

The *property* of a herb refers to its warming or cooling effect on the body. More specifically, herbs are classified according to hot, warm, neutral, cool and cold. As indicated in Chapter 6, these warm and cool properties do not refer to their temperature but the effect on pathogenic heat and cold. Thus peppermint and chrysanthemum are cool, whilst cinnamon and ginseng are warm. Herbs that are hot have stronger effects than warm herbs and can have more serious side effects like internal heat if taken in excess. Examples are *fuzi* and dried ginger. Conversely, herbs that are cold like gypsum and *mudanpi* (made from the root of the peony plant) are used to remove internal heat, but can have the side effects of harming the stomach and spleen if inappropriately used.

The *flavour* of a herb is akin to its taste, except that in Chinese medicine certain actions are associated with the flavour classification, hence there is not always an exact correspondence between flavour and taste. The five flavours are pungent (辛), sweet (甘), sour (酸), bitter (苦) and salty (咸) and their common actions are shown in Table 11.1.

Table 11.1   Five Flavours and Common Actions.

Flavour	Action	Example
Pungent	Dispersing/promoting circulation of *qi* and blood	*Bohe (Herba Mentha)/ Honghua (Flos Carthami)*
Sweet	Nourishing, harmonising and moistening	Ginseng
Sour	Absorbing, consolidating and astringent action	*Wumei* (dried plums)
Bitter	Drying or resolving dampness, purging	*Dahuang* (*Radix et Rhizoma Rhei*)
Salty	Softening hard nodes or masses and promoting defecation	*Mangxiao* (*Natri Sulfas*)

Each herb is thought to have one or more preferential routes along the meridians for their actions to affect specific organs. Chrysanthemum and wolfberry seeds both prefer the liver meridian, and are often used in therapies involving the liver; chrysanthemum also has a preference for the lung meridian and is used in some medications for coughs with heat in the lungs.

11.1.1.2 *Classification by therapeutic effect*

Herbs are also classified according to their principal therapeutic effects. Some of the main classifications are listed below.

1. Diaphoretics (*jiebiao yao* 解表药): removing either warm or cold pathogens at the surface (exterior) level
2. Heat-Clearing (*qingre yao* 清热药): clearing internal heat
3. Purgatives (*xiexia yao* 泻下药): lubricating the large intestine or inducing diarrhoea to move bowels and relieve constipation
4. Removing Dampness (*qushi yao* 祛湿药): eliminating dampness within the body and promoting diuresis
5. Warming Interior (*wenli yao* 温里药): warms interior of body and dispels cold
6. Regulating *Qi* (*liqi yao* 理气药): promoting the movement of *qi*
7. Relieving Food Retention (*xiaoshi yao* 消食药): helps in digestion and relieves food retention
8. Invigorating Blood and Removing Stasis (*huoxue huayu yao* 活血化瘀药): promotes better blood flow and removing stasis
9. Resolving Phlegm (*huatan yao* 化痰药): removing phlegm in the body
10. Tranquilisers (*anshen yao* 安神药): calms the mind

11. Calming Liver and Wind (*pinggan xifeng yao* 平肝熄风药): calming the liver and suppressing hyperactive *yang*, or calming liver-wind
12. Tonics (Restoratives) (*buyi yao* 补益药): tonics for *qi*, blood, *yin* and *yang*
13. Astringents (*shoulian guse yao* 收敛固涩药): arresting excessive discharge of fluids such as perspiration, diarrhoea and urine
14. Hemostatic Herbs (*zhixue yao* 止血药): these assist in stopping bleeding internally and externally, be cooling the blood, warming the channels, or astringent action
15. Eliminating parasites (*shachong yao* 杀虫药)

Although a herb may be classified according to its main action, most herbs have several other actions. This is because a herb contains a large variety of components and molecules, and its action cannot be captured by just one classification. For example, wolfberry seeds or *Gouqizi* (枸杞子) has the main therapeutic effect of tonifying the *yin* of the liver and kidney; it also improves the eyesight and nourishes the lung.

A list of common herbs with descriptions of their nature, properties and principal applications is provided in Annex 1 to this chapter.

11.2 Medical Prescriptions (方剂)

Fangji (方剂) is the TCM term for a medical formulation or prescription. The word *fang* (方) means 'method'; in ordinary language, *youfang* (有方) means having the right method, or the correct approach, to a problem. *Ji* means medicine; hence *fangji* denotes medicine formulated by a good method, i.e. a good prescription.

Chinese physicians have found over the years that herbs can be combined in a certain way to achieve the best desired result; much like a cocktail has a combination of ingredients to yield the best taste, or a food recipe to give us an appetising and nutritious dish. Unlike Western medicine, Chinese prescriptions are customised for the individual, taking into account the type and severity of his syndromes as well as his constitution and state of health.

However, Chinese medicine has over thousands of years also developed a large number of standard prescriptions that can be used for patients falling within a category of syndromes. In practice, these standard or classical prescriptions can and often are modified by the physician to suit the individual. The standard prescriptions are classified by therapeutic effect, similar to the way herbs are classified. Because the prescriptions contain several herbs, each playing a different role, a better result is usually obtained than by using just one herb. This is in contrast to Western drugs, which generally contain one active chemical ingredient with other ingredients only providing a base for the delivery of that active ingredient; to deal with co-morbidities, a number of drugs would be taken together.

The general principle for combining herbs in Chinese medicine is based on one of four possible roles that each herb can play, namely the monarch, ministerial, adjuvant and guiding roles, known as *jun* (君), *chen* (臣), *zuo* (佐), *shi* (使) respectively.

1. The Monarch or *jun* herb plays the core therapeutic role.
2. The Ministerial or *chen* herb enhances the latter's effect.
3. The Adjuvant or *zuo* herb plays a complementary role, supporting the monarch herb by working on a related concomitant condition, or reducing toxicities and side effects, if any, of the monarch and ministerial herbs.
4. The Guiding or *shi* herb helps direct the other herbs to the particular organs and harmonises their joint action.

11.2.1 *Examples of common formulations*

11.2.1.1 *Decoction of the Four Noble Herbs* (*Sijunzi Tang* 四君子汤)

This classical prescription contains ginseng (monarch herb), *baizhu* 白术 (minister herb), *fuling* 茯苓 (adjuvant herb) and *zhigancao* 炙甘草 (guiding herb). A common tonic for the spleen and stomach, this prescription replenishes *qi* and strengthens the spleen. It takes into account that spleen problems are usually accompanied by dampness. In this prescription, ginseng is a strong *qi* tonic, *bai zhu* is also a *qi* tonic that enhances ginseng's *qi*-replenishing action, whilst *fuling* both adds to the *qi* tonic effect and removes dampness. *Zhigancao* harmonises the combination; it is also in itself a mild *qi* and spleen tonic.

Extensions: The formulation can be extended to form related prescriptions for the same family of ailments but with different therapeutic emphasis. For example, the herbs *Pericarpium Citri Tangerinae* (*chenpi* 陈皮) and *Rhizoma Pinellieae* (*banxia* 半夏) can be added to form the Decoction of the Six Noble Herbs (*Liujunzi Tang* 六君子汤). *Chenpi* regulates *qi* and *banxia* resolves phlegm and dampness, hence the addition of these two herbs strengthen the ability of this formulation to relieve dampness and phlegm in the spleen, a condition that frequently develops from weak spleen *qi* that allows dampness pathogen to take hold, causing dyspepsia and nausea. When there is also cold dampness and *qi* flow is impeded, causing a bloated abdomen, lassitude and vomiting, a further two herbs *Fructus Amomi* (*sharen* 砂仁) and *Radix Aucklandiae* (*muxiang* 木香) are added to add strength to removing dampness and regulate *qi* respectively. The formulation has the resolution of dampness as its main objective, buttressed in this action by *qi*-tonifying herbs.

11.2.1.2 *Pill of six ingredients with Rehmanniae (Liuwei Dihuang Wan* 六味地黄丸*)*

Not every prescription has herbs playing all the four roles in combination. Many prescriptions have two or more herbs playing same role. The renowned 'Pill of Six Ingredients with *Rehmanniae* or *Liuwei Dihuang Wan,* a popular *yin* tonic for nourishing the kidney, comprises one monarch herb (*rehmannaie* or *shudihuang* 熟地黄), two ministerial herbs (*shanzhuyu* 山茱萸 and *shanyao* 山药) and three adjuvant herbs (*zexie* 泽泻, *mudanpi* 牡丹皮 and *fuling* 茯苓). The monarch herb is a strong kidney tonic, whilst the two ministerial herbs also nourish the kidney with *shanyao* also strengthening the spleen to complement the kidney function. The three adjuvant herbs play varying roles of reducing dampness, clearing heat arising from *yin* deficiency of the kidney and improving the transportation and transformation function of the spleen. In combination, they tonify the kidney and spleen as well as dissipate internal heat in a balanced and gentle manner, making it one of the most successful prescriptions in the history of Chinese medicine, used equally by physicians treating illnesses, as well as the common man as a dietary supplement to combat the weakening of the kidney functions that come with ageing and with daily stresses.

Extensions: *Liuwei Dihuang Wan* can be modified to treat kidney-*yang* deficiency by adding internal warming herbs like cinnamon (*guizhi* 桂枝) and *Radix Aconite Lateralis Praeparata* (*fuzi* 附子) to form the classic prescription 'Pill for Invigorating Kidney Qi' (*Shenqi Wan* 肾气丸), popular with ageing males with poor libido, dribbling urine, sore backs and aversion to cold. For patients with liver-*yin* weakness and accompanying blurry vision, wolfberry seeds (*gouqizi* 枸杞子) and chrysanthemum (*juhua* 菊花) are added to *Liuwei Dihuang Wan* to form *Qiju Dihuang Wan* 杞菊地黄丸.

11.2.1.3 *Decoction of Gastrodia and Uncaria* (*Tianma Gouteng Yin* 天麻钩藤饮)

This widely used prescription for calming the liver to stop endogenous wind, clearing heat and promoting blood circulation is applied mainly to the treatment of hypertension and post-stroke management of blood pressure. It addresses the syndrome of hyperactive liver-*yang* (*ganyang shangkang* 肝阳上亢) and upward movement of liver wind (*ganfeng shangshao* 肝风上饶) manifested as hypertension with headache and insomnia. It comprises 12 herbs, of which the 6 main ones are listed in Table 10.2.

Tianma and *gouteng* are the monarch herbs, performing the main role expelling liver wind, while *shijueming* and *chuanniuxi* are minister drugs, suppressing a hyperactive *yang* and while also assisting in expelling liver wind. The other herbs serve adjuvant roles, with *huangqin* and *zhizi* clearing heat from the liver meridian.

Table 10.2   Six Main Herbs in *Tianma Gouteng Yin.*

Tianma 天麻	*Rhizoma Gastrodiae*
Gouteng 钩藤	*Ramulus Uncariae cum Uncis*
Shijueming 石决明	*Concha Haliotidis*
Zhizi 栀子	*Fructus Gardeniae*
Huangqin 黄芩	*Radix Scutellariae*
Chuanniuxi 川牛膝	*Radix Archyranthis Bidentatae*

11.2.1.4 *On cocktails and combinations*

Scientist David Ho refers to Chinese herbs as a rich source of drugs, employing an extension of Chinese formulation theory to invent the drugs cocktail concept for his award-winning work on AIDs medications.[226] Ho recounts:

> HIV changes every time it replicates, so high replication rate meant high error rate and therefore HIV was able to mutate very quickly […] if you treat this virus with one or two drugs at a time the virus is predictably going to mutate and escape from the action of the drugs. But at the same time we could also calculate what it would take to corner the virus so it's not able to escape. Those calculations suggested to us that three or more drugs would do the trick. So we knew that by 1995 and launched a series of experiments in patients using what is now called a cocktail therapy of three drugs or more.[227]

The combination of various drugs is reminiscent of the principle of the Chinese prescription, for which there is typically one main (monarch) herb with others supporting it in various distinct roles to form an effective team to fight the prevailing syndromes.

Chinese prescriptions can also be combined as multiple-formulation cocktails. As each standard prescription is targeted at a particular syndrome, patients with multiple syndromes can have several standard formulations combined into one, with suitable adjustments to avoid duplication of herbs that are used in common as well as modifications that reflect the syndrome that is being treated as priority (with larger proportions of the

---

[226] Ho (2001).

[227] David Ho interview (April 20, 2010). http://bigthink.com/videos/discovering-the-hivaids-drug-cocktail-in-an-equation.

ingredients aimed at that syndrome) and the other syndromes which are treated more gently. The choice of such prescriptions for a particular patient at a given time requires judgment and experience and, in a sense, is both a science and art, in some respects like a culinary recipe. It also reinforces the idea that TCM is patient-centric medicine. This has sometimes been compared to Western medicine that is allegedly disease-centric, except for "great" physicians who, according to the noted British-Canadian doctor William Osler, have learnt "to treat the patient who has the disease."[228]

A list of commonly-used prescriptions may be found in Annex 2 to this chapter.

---

[228] The noted British-Canadian physician William Osler noted that "The good physician treats the disease; the great physician treats the patient who has the disease." This reflects a philosophy close to the Chinese tradition of patient-centric customised medications. See "Oslerisms" http://lifeinthefastlane.com/resources/oslerisms/

Annex 1[229]: Common Chinese Herbs

	Diaphoretic Herbs with Pungent Warm Property 辛温解表药		
Name of Herb	Flavour and Nature	Meridian Tropism	Actions
Mahuang 麻黄 (Ephedra)	Pungent and slightly bitter; Warm	Lung and bladder	1. Induce sweating to relieve superficies 2. Ventilate the lung to relieve asthma 3. Promote diuresis
Guizhi 桂枝 (Cinnamon)	Pungent and sweet; Warm	Heart, lung and bladder	1. Induce sweating to relieve superficies 2. Reinforce *yang* and warm the meridians
Fangfeng 防风 (Divaricate Saposhnikovia Root)	Pungent and sweet; Slightly warm	Bladder, liver and spleen	1. Expel wind 2. Resolve dampness to relieve pain 3. Relieve spasms
Shengjiang 生姜 (Fresh Ginger)	Pungent; Warm	Lung, spleen and stomach	1. Expel wind-cold pathogens 2. Warm the abdomen to relieve nausea and vomiting 3. Warm the lung to relieve cough
Xinyi 辛夷 (Magnolia Biondii Flower)	Pungent; Warm	Lung and stomach	1. Expel wind-cold pathogen 2. Clear the nasal passageway
Cangerzi 苍耳子 (Siberian Cocklebur Fruit)	Pungent and bitter; Warm; Slightly toxic	Lung	1. Expel wind-cold pathogen 2. Clear the nasal passageway 3. Dispel wind-dampness 4. Relieve pain

[229] Annexes 1 and 2 were compiled with the assistance of Karen Wee, TCM physician at the Renhai clinic (www.renhai.com.sg).

Diaphoretic Herbs with Pungent Cool Property 辛凉解表药

Name of Herb	Flavour and Nature	Meridian Tropism	Actions
Chaihu 柴胡 (Chinese Thorowax Root)	Pungent and bitter; Slightly cold	Liver and gall bladder	1. Relieve exterior syndrome 2. Anti-pyretic 3. Regulate stagnation of liver-qi 4. Uplift yang-qi
Juhua 菊花 (Chrysanthemum flower)	Pungent, bitter and sweet; Slightly cold	Lung and liver	1. Expel wind-heat 2. Clear liver heat to improve vision 3. Calm and suppress liver-yang 4. Eliminate toxins
Sangye 桑叶 (Mulberry Leaf)	Sweet and bitter; Cold	Lung and liver	1. Expel wind-heat 2. Clear lung-heat and nourish dryness 3. Calm and suppress liver-yang 4. Clear liver-heat to improve vision
Bohe 薄荷 (Peppermint Leaf)	Pungent; Cool	Lung and liver	1. Expel wind-heat from the head, eye and throat 2. Soothe liver and regulate liver-qi stagnation
Gegen 葛根 (Kudzuvine Root)	Pungent and sweet; Cool	Spleen and stomach	1. Anti-pyretic 2. Promote production of fluids to quench thirst 3. Uplift yang-qi to stop diarrhoea 4. Promote the outburst of measles

Herbs for Clearing Heat and Purging Fire 清热泻火药			
Name of Herb	Flavour and Nature	Meridian Tropism	Actions
Shigao 石膏 (Gypsum)	Sweet and pungent; Very cold	Lung and stomach	Raw form 1. Clear heat and purge fire 2. Remove vexation and quench thirst Calcinated form: Stop bleeding and promote the growth of tissue (for treating ulcers)
Zhimu 知母 (Anemarrhena Rhizome)	Bitter and sweet; Cold	Lung, stomach and kidney	1. Clear heat and purge fire 2. Promote the production of fluids for moistening
Danzhuye 淡竹叶 (Lophatherum Herb)	Sweet and bland; Cold	Heart, stomach and small intestine	1. Clear heat and purge fire 2. Relieve vexation 3. Promote diuresis
Zhizi 栀子 (Cape Jasmine Fruit)	Bitter; Cold	Heart, lung and triple energiser	1. Purge fire to remove vexation 2. Clear heat-dampness 3. Cool the blood and eliminate toxins. Charred form can stop bleeding
Xiakucao 夏枯草 (Common Selfheal Fruit-Spike)	Pungent and bitter; Cold	Liver and gall bladder	1. Clear heart and purge fire to improve vision 2. Disperse abnormal growth/masses to reduce swelling
Juemingzi 决明子 (Cassia Seeds)	Sweet, bitter and salty; Slightly cold	Liver and large intestine	1. Clear liver-heat to improve vision 2. Moisten the large intestine to promote bowel movement

Herbs for Clearing Heat-Dampness 清热燥湿药

Name of Herb	Flavour and Nature	Meridian Tropism	Actions
Huangqin 黄芩 (Baical Skullcap Root/ *Radix Scutellariae*)	Bitter; Cold	Lung, gall bladder, spleen, stomach, large and small intestine	1. Clear heat and dry dampness 2. Purge fire and eliminate toxins 3. Stop bleeding 4. Prevent miscarriage
Kushen 苦参 (Light-yellow Sophora Root)	Bitter; Cold	Heart, liver, stomach, large intestine and bladder	1. Clear heat and dry dampness 2. Kill parasites, fungus 3. Promote diuresis

Herbs for Clearing Heat and Eliminating Toxins 清热解毒药

Name of Herb	Flavour and Nature	Meridian Tropism	Actions
Jinyinhua 金银花 (Honeysuckle Flower)	Sweet; Cold	Lung, heart and stomach	1. Eliminate heat and toxins 2. Expel wind-heat pathogens
Lianqiao 连翘 (Weeping Forsythia Capsule)	Bitter; Slightly cold	Lung, heart and small intestine	1. Eliminate heat and toxins 2. Disperse masses/abnormal growth to reduce swelling 3. Expel wind-heat pathogens
Chuanxinlian 穿心莲 (Common Andrographis Herb)	Bitter; Cold	Lung, heart, large intestine and bladder	1. Eliminate heat and toxins 2. Cool the blood 3. Reduce swelling 4. Resolve dampness

(Continued)

(*Continued*)

Herbs for Clearing Heat and Eliminating Toxins 清热解毒药

Name of Herb	Flavour and Nature	Meridian Tropism	Actions
Banlangen 板蓝根 (Isatis root)	Bitter; Cold	Lung and stomach	1. Eliminate heat and toxins 2. Cool the blood 3. Soothe the throat
Yuxingcao 鱼腥草 (Heartleaf Houttuynia)	Pungent; Slightly cold	Lung	1. Eliminate heat and toxins 2. Reduce abscess by promoting pus discharge 3. Remove dampness by promoting diuresis
Machixian 马齿苋 (Purslane)	Sour; Cold	Liver and large intestine	1. Eliminate heat and toxins 2. Cool the blood to stop bleeding 3. Stop dysentry
Pugongyin 蒲公英 (Dandelion)	Bitter and sweet; Cold	Liver and stomach	1. Eliminate heat and toxins 2. Disperse abnormal growth/masses to reduce swelling 3. Promote diuresis
Banbianlian 半边莲	Pungent; Neutral	Heart, lung and small intestine	1. Eliminate heat and toxins 2. Promote diuresis to relieve edema
Baihua Sheshecao 白花蛇舌草 (Oldenlandia)	Sweet and slightly bitter; Cold	Stomach, large and small intestine	1. Eliminate heat and toxins 2. Remove dampness by promoting diuresis

Heat-Clearing and Blood-Cooling Herbs 清热凉血药			
Name of Herb	**Flavour and Nature**	**Meridian Tropism**	**Actions**
Xuanshen 玄参 (Figwort Root)	Sweet, salty and bitter; Slightly cold	Lung, stomach and kidney	1. Clear heat and cool the blood 2. Purge fire and remove toxins 3. Nourish *yin*
Mudanpi 牡丹皮 (Tree Peony Root)	Bitter and sweet; Slightly cold	Heart, liver and kidney	1. Clear heat and cool the blood 2. Promote blood flow and remove stasis
Shengdihuang 生地黄 (Raw Rehmannia Root)	Sweet and bitter; Cold	Heart, liver and kidney	1. Clear heat and cool the blood 2. Nourish *yin* and promote the production of fluids

Herbs for Clearing Asthenic Heat 清虚热药			
Name of Herb	**Flavour and Nature**	**Meridian Tropism**	**Actions**
Qinghao 青蒿 (Sweet wormwood)	Bitter and pungent; Cold	Liver and gall bladder	1. Clear asthenic heat and summer heat 2. Cool the blood 3. Treat malaria

Purgatives 泻下药			
Name of Herb	**Flavour and Nature**	**Meridian Tropism**	**Actions**
Dahuang 大黄 (Rhubarb)	Bitter; Cold	Spleen, stomach, large intestine, liver and pericardium	1. Promote bowel movement by clearing heat and purging fire 2. Cool blood and remove toxins 3. Remove blood stasis
Fanxieye 番泻叶 (Senna Leaf)	Sweet and bitter; Cold	Large intestine	Purge to promote bowel movement
Huomaren 火麻仁 (Hemp Seed)	Sweet; Neutral	Spleen, stomach and large intestine	Promote bowel movement by moistening the intestine

Herbs for Resolving Dampness 化湿药

Name of Herb	Flavour and Nature	Meridian Tropism	Actions
Huoxiang 藿香 (Cablin Patchouli Herb)	Pungent; Slightly warm	Spleen, stomach and lung	1. Resolve dampness 2. Relieve nausea and vomiting 3. Clear summer-heat
Cangzhu 苍术 (Atractylodes Rhizome)	Pungent and bitter; Warm	Spleen, stomach and liver	1. Dry dampness and strengthen the spleen 2. Expel wind and disperse the cold
Houpo 厚朴 (Official Magnolia Bark)	Pungent and bitter; Warm	Spleen, stomach, lung and large intestine	1. Dry dampness and resolve phlegm 2. Promote the descent of *qi* to remove stagnation
Sharen 砂仁 (Villous Amomum Fruit)	Pungent; Warm	Spleen, stomach and kidney	1. Resolve dampness and regulate *qi* 2. Warm the abdomen and stop diarrhoea 3. Prevent miscarriage
Doukou 豆蔻 (Cardamon Fruit)	Pungent; Warm	Spleen, stomach and lung	1. Resolve dampness and regulate *qi* 2. Warm the abdomen to relieve nausea and vomiting

Herbs for Removing Wind-Dampness 祛风湿药

Name of Herb	Flavour and Nature	Meridian Tropism	Actions
Wujiapi 五加皮 (Slenderstyle Acanthopanax Bark)	Pungent and bitter; Warm	Liver and kidney	1. Remove wind-dampness 2. Tonify the liver and kidney 3. Strengthen the ligaments and bone 4. Promote diuresis

Diuretics 利水渗湿药

Name of Herb	Flavour and Nature	Meridian Tropism	Actions
Fuling 茯苓 (Poria)	Sweet and bland; Neutral	Heart, spleen and kidney	1. Promote diuresis to drain dampness and relieve edema 2. Invigorate spleen 3. Tranquilise the mind
Yiyiren 薏苡仁 (Job's Tears)	Sweet and bland; Cool	Spleen, stomach and lung	1. Promote diuresis to drain dampness and relieve edema 2. Invigorate spleen 3. Relieve joint pain 4. Clear heat and promote pus discharge
Dongguaren 冬瓜仁 (Winter melon seeds)	Sweet; Cool	Spleen and small intestine	1. Clear lung-heat and resolve phlegm 2. Remove dampness and promote pus discharge

Herbs for Regulating Qi 理气药

Name of Herb	Flavour and Nature	Meridian Tropism	Actions
Chenpi 陈皮 (Dried tangerine peel)	Pungent and bitter; Warm	Spleen and lung	1. Regulate *qi* and invigorate spleen 2. Dry dampness and resolve phlegm
Xiangfu 香附 (Nutgrass Galingale Rhizome)	Pungent, slightly bitter and sweet; Neutral	Liver, spleen and triple energiser	1. Regulate liver-*qi* stagnation 2. Regulate menstruation and relieve pain 3. Regulate spleen and stomach-*qi*
Meiguihua 玫瑰花 (Rose flower)	Sweet and slightly bitter; Warm	Spleen and liver	1. Regulate liver-*qi* stagnation 2. Promote blood flow to relieve pain

Herbs for Promoting Digestion 消食药

Name of Herb	Flavour and Nature	Meridian Tropism	Actions
Shanzha 山楂 (Hawthorn Berry)	Sweet and sour; Slightly warm	Spleen, stomach and liver	1. Promote digestion 2. Regulate *qi* and remove stasis
Maiya 麦芽 (Germinated Barley)	Sweet; Neutral	Spleen, stomach and liver	1. Promote digestion and strengthen the stomach 2. Promote lactation
Laifuzi 莱菔子 (Radish seed)	Sweet and pungent; Neutral	Spleen, stomach and lung	1. Promote digestion and relieve abdomen distension 2. Promote the descent of *qi* and resolve dampness

Interior Warming Herbs 温里药

Name of Herb	Flavour and Nature	Meridian Tropism	Actions
Fuzi 附子 (Lateralis Preparata)	Pungent and sweet; Very Hot; Toxic	Heart, spleen and kidney	1. Restore *yang* (for severe deficiency of *yang*) 2. Strengthen *yang* by restoring fire 3. Disperse cold to alleviate pain
Ganjiang 干姜 (Zingiber Dried Ginger)	Pungent; Hot	Spleen, stomach, kidney, heart and lung	1. Warm the abdomen and disperse cold 2. Restore *yang* to warm and clear the collaterals 3. Warm the lung to resolve rheum
Rougui 肉桂 (Cassia Bark)	Pungent and sweet; Very Hot	Kidney, spleen, heart and liver	1. Strengthen *yang* by restoring fire 2. Disperse cold to alleviate pain 3. Warm the meridians to clear the collaterals 4. Return fire to the origin (kidney)
Huajiao 花椒 (Pricklyash Peel)	Pungent; Warm	Spleen, stomach and kidney	1. Warm the abdomen to relieve pain 2. Kill parasites to relieve itching

Hemostatics 止血药

Name of Herb	Flavour and Nature	Meridian Tropism	Actions
Sanqi 三七	Sweet and slightly bitter; Warm	Liver and stomach	1. Remove blood stasis to stop bleeding 2. Promote blood circulation to relieve pain

Herbs for Promoting Blood Circulation and Removing Stasis 活血化瘀药

Name of Herb	Flavour and Nature	Meridian Tropism	Actions
Chuanxiong 川芎 (Szechwan Lovage Rhizome)	Pungent; Warm	Liver, gall bladder and pericardium	1. Promote blood circulation and regulate *qi* 2. Expel wind to relieve pain
Jianghuang 姜黄 (Tumeric)	Pungent and bitter; Warm	Spleen and liver	1. Promote blood circulation and regulate *qi* 2. Clear the collaterals to relieve pain
Moyao 没药 (Myrrh)	Pungent and bitter; Neutral	Heart, liver and spleen	1. Promote blood circulation to relieve pain 2. Reduce swelling and promote healing
Danshen 丹参	Bitter; Slightly cold	Heart, pericardium, and liver	1. Promote blood circulation to regulate menstruation 2. Remove stasis to relieve pain 3. Cool the blood to promote the healing of carbuncle 4. Remove vexation and calm the mind
Honghua 红花 (Safflower)	Bitter and sweet; Neutral	Heart, liver and large intestine	1. Promote blood circulation and remove stasis 2. Moisten the large intestine to promote bowel movement 3. Relieve cough and dyspnea
Taoren 桃仁 (Peach Seed)	Pungent; Warm; Slightly toxic	Heart and liver	1. Promote blood circulation and menstruation 2. Remove blood stasis to relieve pain

Herbs for Resolving Phlegm and Relieving Cough and Dyspnea 止咳化痰平喘 药

Name of Herb	Flavour and Nature	Meridian Tropism	Actions
Banxia 半夏 (Pinellia Tuber)	Pungent; Warm; Toxic	Spleen, stomach and lung	1. Dry dampness and resolve phlegm 2. Relieve nausea and vomiting by suppressing the adverse rise of *qi* 3. Relieve abdominal distension and disperse masses
Jiegeng 桔梗 (Hogfennel Root)	Bitter and pungent; Neutral	Lung	1. Disperse lung-*qi* 2. Expel phlegm 3. Soothe the throat 4. Promote the discharge of pus
Gualou 瓜蒌 (Snakegourd Fruit)	Sweet and slightly bitter; Cold	Lung, stomach and large intestine	1. Clear heat and resolve phlegm 2. Regulate *qi* stagnation in the chest and disperse abnormal masses/growths 3. Moisten the large intestine to promote bowel movement
Chuanbeimu 川贝母 (Tendrilleaf Fritillary Bulb)	Bitter and Sweet; Slightly cold	Lung and heart	1. Clear heat and resolve phlegm 2. Moisten the lung to relieve cough 3. Disperse abnormal masses or growths to reduce swelling
Zhebeimu 浙贝母 (Thunberg Fritillary Bulb)	Bitter; Cold	Lung and heart	1. Clear heat and resolve phlegm 2. Disperse abnormal masses or growths to promote healing of carbuncle

(*Continued*)

(Continued)

Herbs for Resolving Phlegm and Relieving Cough and Dyspnea 止咳化痰平喘药

Name of Herb	Flavour and Nature	Meridian Tropism	Actions
Luohanguo 罗汉果	Sweet; Cool	Lung and large intestine	1. Clear heat from the lung and soothe the throat 2. Resolve phlegm and relieve cough 3. Moisten the large intestine to promote bowel movement
Kuxingren 苦杏仁 (Bitter Almond Seed)	Bitter; Slightly warm; Slightly toxic	Lung and large intestine	1. Relieve cough and dyspnea 2. Moisten the large intestine to promote bowel movement
Ziyuan 紫菀 (Tatarian Aster Root)	Bitter, sweet and pungent; Slightly warm	Lung	1. Moisten the lung and resolve phlegm to relieve cough
Kuandonghua 款冬花 (Common Clotsfoot Flower)	Pungent and slightly bitter; Warm	Lung	1. Moisten the lung, promote the descending of lung-*qi* and resolve phlegm to relieve cough
Pipaye 枇杷叶 (Loquat Leaf)	Bitter; Slightly cold	Lung and stomach	1. Clear lung heat to relieve cough 2. Promote the descent of *qi* to relieve nausea and vomiting
Baiguo 白果 (Gingko Seed)	Sweet, bitter and astringent; Neutral; Toxic	Lung	1. Astringe lung and resolve phlegm to relieve dyspnea 2. Stop abnormal vagina discharge (leucorrhoea) and reduce urination

	Calmatives 安神药		
Name of Herb	Flavour and Nature	Meridian Tropism	Actions
Longgu 龙骨 (Dragon Bone)	Sweet and astringent; Neutral	Heart, lung and kidney	1. Tranquilise the mind 2. Calm the liver to suppress liver-*yang* 3. Arrest fluids (calcinated form)
Suanzaoren 酸枣仁 (Spine Date Seed)	Sour and sweet; Neutral	Heart, liver and gall bladder	1. Nourish the heart and liver 2. Calm the mind 3. Arrest sweating
Yejiaoteng 夜交藤	Sweet; Neutral	Heart and liver	1. Nourish the blood to calm the mind 2. Expel wind to clear the collaterals
Baiziren 柏子仁 (Chinese Arborvitae Kernel)	Sweet; Neutral	Heart, kidney and large intestine	1. Nourish the heart to calm the mind 2. Moisten the intestine to promote bowel movement
Hehuanpi 合欢皮 (Silktree Albizia Bark)	Sweet; Neutral	Heart, liver and lung	1. Alleviate depression to calm the mind 2. Promote blood circulation to relieve swelling
Lingzhi 灵芝 (Lucid Ganoderma)	Sweet; Neutral	Heart, lung, liver and kidney	1. Strengthen *qi* to calm the mind 2. Relieve cough and asthma

Qi Tonics 补气药

Name of Herb	Flavour and Nature	Meridian Tropism	Actions
Renshen 人参 (Ginseng)	Sweet, Slightly bitter; Neutral	Lung, spleen and heart	1. Invigorate *qi* 2. Tonify the spleen and strengthen the lung 3. Promote the production of fluids 4. Calm the nerves for better concentration and also sounder sleep
Xiyangshen 西洋参 (American Ginseng)	Sweet, Slightly bitter; Cool	Lung, heart, kidney and spleen	1. Invigorate *qi* and nourish *yin* 2. Clear heat and promote the production of fluids
Dangshen 党参 (Tangshen)	Sweet; Neutral	Spleen and lung	1. Invigorate the spleen and lung functions by tonifying their *qi* 2. Tonify blood 3. Promote the production of fluids
Taizishen 太子参 (Heterophylly Falsestarwort Root)	Sweet, Slightly bitter; Neutral	Spleen and lung	1. Invigorate *qi* and strengthen the spleen functions 2. Promote the production of fluids to moisten the lung
Huangqi 黄芪 (Astragalus)	Sweet; Slightly warm	Spleen and lung	1. Strengthen the spleen functions 2. Uplift *yang-qi* 3. Consolidate the exterior to strengthen the body's defence against external pathogens 4. Promote diuresis and the healing of wounds/ulcers

(Continued)

(*Continued*)

Qi Tonics 补气药

Name of Herb	Flavour and Nature	Meridian Tropism	Actions
Baizhu 白术 (Largehead Astractylodes Rhizome)	Sweet and bvitter; Warm	Spleen and stomach	1. Strengthen spleen and tonify *qi* 2. Dry dampness and promote diuresis 3. Stop perspiration 4. Prevent miscarriage
Shanyao 山药 (Wild Yam)	Sweet; Neutral	Spleen, lung and kidney	1. Tonify the spleen and nourish the stomach 2. Promote the production of fluids and tonify the lung 3. Tonify the kidney 4. Conserve essence
Gancao 甘草 (Liquorice Root)	Sweet; Neutral	Heart, lung, spleen and stomach	1. Tonify the spleen 2. Resolve phlegm and relieve cough 3. Relieve pain 4. Clear heat and eliminate toxins (raw liquorice) 5. Regulate the actions of herbs in a prescription
Dazao 大枣 (Chinese Dates)	Sweet; Warm	Spleen, stomach and heart	1. Strengthen the spleen functions and tonify *qi* 2. Nourish blood to calm the mind
Baibiandou 白扁豆 (White Hyacinth Bean)	Sweet; Slightly warm	Spleen and stomach	1. Tonify the spleen 2. Resolve dampness

Yang Tonics 补阳药

Name of Herb	Flavour and Nature	Meridian Tropism	Actions
Lurong 鹿茸 (Hairy Antler)	Sweet; Warm	Kidney and lung	1. Tonify kidney-*yang* 2. Tonify blood and essence 3. Strengthen the bone and tendons 4. Regulate the *chong* 冲 and *ren* 任 vessels (they govern the menstruation) 5. Promote the healing of sores/ulcers
Yinyanghuo 淫羊藿 (Horny-goat Weed)	Pungent and sweet; Warm	Kidney and liver	1. Tonify the kidney and boost *yang* 2. Expel wind and remove dampness
Duzhong 杜仲 (Eucommia Bark)	Sweet; Warm	Liver and kidney	1. Tonify the kidney and liver 2. Strengthen the bones and tendons 3. Prevent miscarriage
Dongchongxiacao 冬虫夏草 (Cordyceps)	Sweet and salty; Warm	Kidney and lung	1. Tonify the kidney and lung 2. Resolve phlegm 3. Stop bleeding
Hetaoren 核桃仁 (Walnut)	Sweet; Warm	Kidney, lung and large intestine	1. Tonify the kidney and warm the lung 2. Moisten the large intestine to promote bowel movement

Blood Tonics 补血药			
Name of Herb	**Flavour and Nature**	**Meridian Tropism**	**Actions**
Shudihuang 熟地黄 (Processed Rehmannia Root)	Sweet; Slightly warm	Liver and kidney	1. Tonify blood and nourish *yin* 2. Supplement essence and marrow
Ejiao 阿胶 (Equus asinus Linnaeus)	Sweet; Neutral	Lung, liver and kidney	1. Tonify blood and nourish *yin* 2. Moisten the lung 3. Stop bleeding
Heshouwu 何首乌 (Fleeceflower Root)	Bitter, sweet, astringent; Slightly warm	Kidney and liver	Processed form: 1. Tonify and enrich blood Raw form: 1. Eliminate toxins 2. Treat malaria 3. Moisten the large intestine to promote bowel movement
Longyanrou 龙眼肉 (Logan Meat)	Sweet; Warm	Heart and spleen	1. Tonify the heart and spleen 2. Nourish blood to calm the mind
Danggui 当归 (Chinese Angelica)	Sweet and pungent; Warm	Liver, heart and spleen	1. Tonify blood and regulate menstruation 2. Promote blood circulation to relieve pain 3. Moisten the large intestine to promote bowel movement

Yin Tonics 补阴药

Name of Herb	Flavour and Nature	Meridian Tropism	Actions
Beishashen 北沙参 (Coastal Glehnia Root)	Sweet and slightly bitter; Slightly cold	Lung and stomach	1. Nourish lung-*yin* and clear lung heat 2. Tonify the stomach and promote the production of fluids
Baihe 百合 (Lily Bulb)	Sweet; Slightly cold	Lung, heart and stomach	1. Nourish *yin* and moisten the lung 2. Clear heat from the heart to calm the mind
Maidong 麦冬 (Dwarf Lilyturf Tuber)	Sweet and slightly bitter; Slightly cold	Lung, stomach and heart	1. Nourish *yin* and promote the production of fluids 2. Moisten the lung 3. Clear heat from the heart
Shihu 石斛 (Dendrobium)	Sweet; Slightly cold	Stomach and kidney	1. Tonify the stomach and promote the production of fluids 2. Nourish *yin* and clear asthenic heat
Yuzhu 玉竹 (Fragrant Solomonseal Rhizome)	Sweet; Slightly cold	Lung and stomach	1. Nourish *yin* and moisten dryness 2. Promote the production of fluids to quench thirst
Gouqizi 枸杞子 (Wolfberry Seed)	Sweet; Neutral	Liver and kidney	1. Nourish and tonify the kidney and liver 2. Tonify essence and improve vision
Guijia 龟甲 (Tortise Shell)	Sweet; Cold	Liver, kidney and heart	1. Nourish *yin* and suppress *yang* 2. Tonify kidney and strengthen bone 3. Nourish blood and tonify the heart
Heizhima 黑芝麻 (Black Sesame Seed)	Sweet; Neutral	Liver, kidney and large intestine	1. Tonify the kidney and liver 2. Moisten the large intestine 3. Tonify essence and blood

Astringent Herbs 收涩药

Name of Herb	Flavour and Nature	Meridian Tropism	Actions
Wuweizi 五味子 (Chinese Magnoliavine Fruit)	Sour and sweet; Slightly warm	Lung, heart and kidney	1. Reduce sweating 2. Calm the mind 3. Tonify the kidney 4. Tonify *qi* and promote the production of fluids
Lianzi 莲子 (Lotus seed)	Sweet and astringent; Neutral	Spleen, heart and kidney	1. Prevent abnormal discharge and involuntary seminal emission 2. Tonify the spleen to relieve diarrhoea 3. Tonify the kidney 4. Calm the mind by nourishing the heart

Annex 2: Common Chinese Prescriptions

The prescriptions listed below are representative of the various formulations categorised by their principal therapeutic functions. The Chinese names are provided and, where commonly used, the English translations as well. Each prescription typically ends with 'san' if it is usually prepared as a powder, 'yin' or 'tang' if it is a decoction and 'wan' if in pill form. In practice, most decoctions are also available in pharmacies in the form of pills, tablets or capsules as these are more convenient for daily use.

	Diaphoretic Prescriptions	
1	Yinqiaosan 银翘散	Expels wind-heat exogenous pathogens. Eliminates heat and toxins. Often used in the early stage of an external syndrome invaded by wind-heat pathogens.
2	Guizhitang 桂枝汤	Expels wind-cold exogenous pathogens. Regulates the nutrient and defensive *qi* to strengthen the body. Can be used for treating external syndromes caused by wind-cold exogenous pathogens or for individuals who feel weak and are recovering from chronic illnesses.
	Prescriptions for Clearing Internal Heat	
3	Daochisan 导赤散	Clears heat from the heart. Promotes diuresis and nourishes *yin*. Treats the syndrome of exuberance of heart fire.
4	Longdan Xiegan Tang 龙胆泻肝汤	Purges fire from the liver and gall bladder. Clears dampness and heat in the lower energiser. Treats sthenic syndrome of the exuberance of liver fire.
5	Yunujian 玉女煎	Clears heat from the stomach and nourishes kidney-*yin*. Treats the syndrome of stomach fire with *yin* deficiency.

(Continued)

	Prescriptions for Removing Dampness	
6	Huoxiang Zhengqi San 藿香正气散	Removes dampness and regulates *qi* in the abdomen region. Used for treating vomiting and diarrhoea caused by cold dampness and wind.
7	Wulingsan 五苓散	Promotes diuresis and removes dampness. Warms *yang-qi* to enhance the function of *qi* to regulate water metabolism. Can be used for treating edema due to retention of water and dampness.
	Prescriptions for Removing Wind-Dampness	
8	Duhuo Jisheng Tang 独活寄生汤	Expels wind-dampness to relieve arthritic pain. Tonifies kidney, liver, *qi* and blood. Treats deficiency syndrome in liver, kidney, *qi* and blood.
9	Danggui Niantong Tang 当归拈痛汤	Drains dampness and clears heat. Expels wind to relieve arthritic pain. Treats damp-heat syndrome.
10	Juanbitang 蠲痹汤	Tonifies *qi* and nourishes blood. Expels wind and dampness. Treats wind-cold-dampness syndrome and relieves arthritic pain.
	Prescriptions for Promoting Digestion	
11	Baohewan 保和丸 'Pill for Preserving Harmony'	Promotes digestion of food. Treats food retention syndrome.
	Prescriptions for Promoting Blood Flow and Removing Blood Stasis	
12	Xuefu Zhuyu Tang 血府逐瘀汤	Promotes blood flow and removes stasis. Regulates *qi* and relieves pain. Often used for treating blood stasis syndrome.

(Continued)

(*Continued*)

	Prescriptions for Resolving Phlegm and Relieving Cough	
13	Qingqi Huatan Tang 清气化痰汤	Clears heat and resolves phlegm. Regulates *qi* and relieves cough. Treats heat-phlegm syndrome.
14	Banxia Houpo Tang 半夏厚朴汤	Regulates *qi* to disperse clumps. Suppresses adverse rise of *qi* and resolves phlegm. Treats 梅核气 *meiheqi* — a feeling of something in the throat that cannot be swallowed or expectorated.
15	Erchen Tang 二陈汤	Removes dampness, resolves phlegm and promotes *qi* flow. Used in wet cough due to phlegm-dampness with white sputum.
	Prescriptions for Calming the Mind	
16	Suanzaoren Tang 酸枣仁汤 'Jujube Seed Decoction'	Nourishes blood and calms the mind. Clears asthenic heat to relieve vexation. Often used to treat insomnia resulting from the deficiency syndrome in liver blood.
17	Tianwang Buxin Dan 天王补心丹	Nourishes *yin* and blood. Tranquilises heart to calm the mind. Treats *yin* deficiency syndrome in the heart and kidney.
	Prescriptions for Regulating the Liver and Spleen	
18	Xiaoyao San 逍遥散 'Ease Powder'	Soothes the liver and regulates the spleen. Used in stagnation of liver-*qi* and deficiency of blood and spleen, with liver suppressing spleen (over-restraint relationship).
19	Danzhi Xiaoyaosan 丹栀逍遥散 (extension of ease powder)	Soothes the liver, regulates *qi* and clears liver fire. Used in liver stagnation stirring up fire.
	Prescriptions for Removing Wind (Both Exogenous and Endogenous Wind)	
20	Tianma Gouteng Yin 天麻钩藤饮	Calms the liver to remove endogenous wind. Clears heat and nourishes liver/kidney. Used for treating headache and dizziness caused by hyperactivity of liver-*yang* syndrome.
21	Xiaofengsan 消风散	Expels wind and nourishes blood. Clears heat and removes dampness. Treats eczema and rubella caused by wind-heat or wind-dampness syndrome.

(*Continued*)

(Continued)

	Prescriptions for Removing Dryness	
22	Qingzao Jiufei Tang 清燥救肺汤	Clears exogenous dry-heat pathogen and moistens the lung. Treats severe syndrome of dryness in the lung.
23	Baihe Gujing Tang 百合固金汤	Nourishes *yin* and moistens lung. Resolves phlegm and relieves cough. Treats cough caused by the deficiency syndrome of kidney and lung-*yin*. (Used in the more advanced stage as the lung-*yin* has been severely damaged.)
	Prescriptions for Tonifying *Qi*	
24	Decoction of the Four Noble Herbs (Sijunzi Tang) 四君子汤	Tonifies *qi* and strengthens spleen. Used in deficiency syndrome of spleen and stomach.
25	Decoction of the Six Noble Herbs 六君子汤 (extension of Decoction of the Four Noble Herbs)	Used for deficiency of spleen/stomach syndrome with dampness and phlegm.
26	Decoction of *Xiangsha Liujunzi Tang* 香砂六君子汤 (extension of Decoction of Six Noble Herbs)	Used for spleen-stomach deficiency with more pronounced dampness and phlegm leading to *qi* stagnation.
27	Shenling Baizhu San 参苓白术散	Tonifies *qi* and strengthens spleen. Resolves dampness. Treats *qi* deficiency syndrome of the spleen and stomach with dampness.
28	Buzhong Yiqi Tang 补中益气汤	Tonifies *qi* and strengthens spleen. Uplifts spleen *yang-qi*. Treats *qi* deficiency syndrome of the spleen and stomach.

(Continued)

(Continued)

29	Yupingfeng San 玉屏风散 (Jade Screen Powder)	Replenishes *qi*, consolidates the superficies and arrests perspiration (reduces sweating). Used in individuals with *qi* deficiency (defensive *qi*).
30	Pulse-activating Powder 生脉饮 (*Shengmai Yin*)	Tonifies *qi* and promotes the production of fluids. Astringes *yin* and arrests sweating. For treatment of deficiency syndrome of *qi* and *yin* resulting in spontaneous sweating and chronic dry cough accompanied by breathlessness, fatigue, etc.
Prescriptions for Tonifying Blood		
31	Decoction of the Four Ingredients 四物汤 (*Siwu Tang)*	Nourishes and regulates blood without introducing stasis. Used in blood deficiency syndrome; Often used for regulating menstruation.
32	Decoction of *Taohong Siwu Tang* 桃红四物汤 (extension of decoction of the four ingredients)	Promotes blood circulation and removes stasis. Used in blood deficiency syndrome with stasis resulting in early menses with blood clots.
33	Chinese Angelica Decoction for Tonifying the Blood 当归补血汤 (Danggui Buxue Tang)	Invigorates *qi* to promote blood production. Used in blood deficiency syndrome, particularly blood deficiency with fever and headache following childbirth or menstrual disorder with severe loss of blood; anemia.
34	Decoction for Restoring the Spleen 归脾汤 (*Guipitang*)	Tonifies *qi* and blood. Strengthens the spleen and nourishes the heart. Treats deficiency syndrome in heart and spleen.
35	Danggui Yinzi 当归饮子	Nourishes blood and promotes its flow. Expels wind to relieve pain. Treats eczema or rubella caused by blood deficiency syndrome (with the invasion of wind pathogen).

(Continued)

(Continued)

Prescriptions for Tonifying *Qi* and Blood		
36	Decoction of the 8 Precious Ingredients 八珍汤	Nourishes *qi* and blood. Used for those with prolonged weakness of *qi* and blood caused by excessive haemorrhage and low *qi* level.
37	Shiquan Dabutang 十全大补汤 'Decoction of 10 Powerful Herbs' (extension of decoction of the 8 precious ingredients)	Warms and tonifies *qi* and blood. Used in deficiency syndrome in *qi* and blood, accompanied by slight *yang* deficiency.
Prescriptions for Tonifying Yang		
38	Pill for Nourishing Kidney-*Yang* (Shenqi Wan) 肾气丸	Warms and invigorates kidney-*yang*. Used to treat deficiency of kidney-*yang* syndrome, often accompanied by weakness of back and knees, coldness in lower trunk, frequent night urination, sexual dysfunction.
39	Jisheng Shenqi Wan 济生肾气丸 (extension of Shenqi Wan)	Warms kidney-*yang* and promotes diuresis to relieve edema. It is often used to treat water retention due to kidney-*yang* deficiency.
Prescriptions for Tonifying Yin		
40	Liuwei Dihuang Wan 六味地黄丸 'Pill of Six Ingredients with Rehmanniae'	Nourishes *yin* and invigorates the kidney. Used in deficiency syndrome of kidney and liver-*yin*, leading to flare up of kidney deficiency fire. Marked by tinnitus, night sweats, emissions, sore throat. Some diabetes patients exhibit such a syndrome.

Bibliography

Akazawa, N *et al.* (2012). Curcumin ingestion and exercise training improve vascular endothelial function in postmenopausal women. *Nutrition Research*, 32(10): 795–799.

Ban, TA (2006). The role of serendipity in drug discovery. *Dialogues Clinical Neuroscience*, 8(3): 335–344.

Bardsley, JL (1845). Diabetes. In: R Dunglison (Ed.) *Encyclopaedia of Practical Medicine*, American Edition, Volume 1, pp. 606–625. Philadelphia: Lea and Blanchard.

Barton, JC (2009). Therapeutic phlebotomy (TP) for hereditary hemochromatosis (HH): A practical guide for patients and health care personnel. *Links on Hemochromatosis*. Retrieved 12 July 2009. http://www.hemochromatosis.co.uk/tp.html.

Becker, S, Flaws, B and Casanas, R (2005). *The Treatment of Cardiovascular Diseases with Chinese Medicine.* Boulder, Colorado: Blue Poppy Press.

Beecher, HK (1955). The powerful placebo. *Journal of the American Medical Association*, 159(17): 1602–1606.

Bensoussan, A. *et al.* (1998). Treatment of irritable bowel syndrome with Chinese herbal medicine: A randomized controlled trial. *Journal of the American Medical Association*, 280(18): 1585–1589.

Bian Zhaoxiang (2010). TCM concepts in the trials. Unpublished paper presented at the *Annual Meeting of the Consortium for the Globalisation of Chinese Medicine (CGCM)*, 24 August 2010.

Brinkhaus, B *et al.* (2006). Acupuncture in patients with chronic low back pain: A randomised controlled trial. *Archives of Internal Medicine*, 166: 450–457.

Buck, C (2000). On terminology. *Journal of Chinese Medicine*, 63: 38–42.

Campbell, N (1920). *Physics: The Elements.* Cambridge: Cambridge University Press.

Campbell, TC and Campbell, TM (2004). *The China Study.* Dallas: Benbella Books.

Carter, KC (2003). *The Rise of the Causal Concepts of Disease.* Ashgate.

Chai Kefu (2007). *Fundamental Theory of Traditional Chinese Medicine.* Beijing: People's Publishing House.

Churchill, W (1999). Implications of evidence based medicine for complementary and alternative medicine. *Journal of Chinese Medicine*, 59: 32–35.

Cullen, C (2001). Yi'an: The origins of a genre of Chinese medical literature. In: E Hsu (Ed.) *Innovation in Chinese Medicine.* Cambridge: Cambridge University Press.

Cumston, CG (1926). *An Introduction to the History of Medicine.* London: Kegan, Paul, Trench, Trubner & Co Ltd.

Damber, JK and Aus, G (2008). Prostate cancer. *The Lancet*, 371(9625): 1710–1721.

DCScience (12 April 2010). More quackedemia. Dangerous Chinese medicine taught at Middlesex University. *DC's Improbably Science.* Retrieved 17 December 2013. http://www.dcscience.net/?p=2923.

Deng Tietao 邓铁涛 (1988). *Lue lun wuzang xiangguan qudai wuxing xueshuo* (On replacing *Wuxing* theory with the theory of five-organ relationships). *Journal of the Guangzhou University of Chinese Medicine*, 2: page range.

Deng Tietao 邓铁涛 (2004). *Yian Yu Yanjiu* 医案与研究 (*Medical Cases for Research*). *Renmin Weisheng Chubanshe* (Publisher).

Daodejing. This classic attributed to Laotze (circa 6th century BC) is widely available. Retrieved 23 December 2013. http://zxuw.cn/daodejng.

Douglas, HE (2009). *Science, Policy, and the Value-Free Ideal,* Pittsburgh.

Edelstein, L (1967). The Methodists. In: O Temkin and CL Temkin (Eds.) *Ancient Medicine: Selected Papers of Ludwig Edelstein*, pp. 173–191. Baltimore: Johns Hopkins University Press.

Ernst, E and White, A (Eds.) (1999). *Acupuncture: A Scientific Appraisal.* Oxford: Butterworth-Heinemann.

Esselstyn, CB (2008). *Prevent and Reverse Heart Disease.* New York: Avery.

Evans, AS (1993). *Causation and Disease: A Chronological Journey.* New York: Plenum Publishing.

Evans, D (2003). *Placebo: The Belief Effect.* Oxford: Harper Collins.

Evans, D (2005). Suppression of the acute-phase response as a biological mechanism for the placebo effect. *Medical Hypotheses,* 64: 1–7.

Fan, RP (2003). Modern Western science as a standard for traditional Chinese medicine: A critical appraisal. *Journal of Law and Medical Ethics,* 31: 213–221.

Fang Zhouzi 方舟子 (2007). *Piping Zhongyi* 批评中医 (*A Critique of Chinese Medicine*). China Xiehe Medical University Press.

Farquhar, J (1994). *Knowing Practice: The Clinical Encounter in Chinese Medicine.* Boulder: Westview Press.

Filshie, J and Cummings, M (1999). Western medical acupuncture. In: E Ernst and A White (Eds.) *Acupuncture: A Scientific Appraisal.* Oxford: Butterworth-Heinemann.

Finniss, D, Kaptchuk, T, Miller, F and Benedett, B (2010). Biological, clinical, and ethical advances of placebo effects, *Lancet,* 375: 686–695.

Forrester, J (1996). If *p*, then what? Thinking in cases. *History of the Human Sciences,* 9(3): 1–25.

Frigg, R and Hartmann, S (2006). Models in science. In: *Stanford Encyclopedia of Philosophy.*

Giere, RN (1988). *Explaining Science.* Chicago: University of Chicago Press.

Giere, RN (1999). *Science Without Laws.* Chicago: University of Chicago Press.

Grmek, MD (Ed.) (1998). *Western Medical Thought from Antiquity to the Middle Ages.* Cambridge: Harvard University Press.

Guo, S *et al.* (2009). Building and evaluating an animal model for syndrome in traditional Chinese medicine in the context of unstable angina (myocardial ischemia) by supervised data mining approaches. *Journal of Biological Systems,* 17(4): 531–546.

Guyatt, G *et al.* (1992). Evidence-based medicine. *Journal of the American Medical Association,* 268: 2420–2425.

Haake, M *et al.* (2007). German Acupuncture Trials (GERAC) for chronic low back pain: Randomised, multicenter, blinded, parallel-group trial with 3 groups. *Archives of Internal Medicine,* 167: 1892–1898.

Hacking, I (1992). Style for historians and philosophers. *Studies in History and Philosophy of Science*, 23: 1–20.

Hanson, M (2001). Robust northerners and delicate southerners: The nineteenth-century invention of a southern *wenbing* tradition. In: E Hsu (Ed.) *Innovation in Chinese Medicine*. Cambridge: Cambridge University Press.

He Jing, 何静 (2005). 从库恩的科学发展模式谈中医学发展的几个问题 (Problems in the development of traditional Chinese medicine from the point of view of Kuhn's model of scientific change). *Journal of the Guizhou College of TCM*, 27(1): 7–10.

He Yuming (2005). 中医方法论 *Treatise on the Methods of Chinese Medicine*. China: *Xiehe* Medical University Press.

Hempel, CG (1966). *Philosophy of Natural Science*. Englewood Cliffs. NJ: Prentice-Hall.

Henle (1844). Medicinische wissenschaft und empire. *Zeitschrift fur rationale Medizin*, 2: 287–412.

Hesse, M. (1967). Models and analogies. In: P Edwards (Ed.) *Encyclopedia of Philosophy*. New York: Macmillan.

Ho, D (2001). Taiwanese scientist to test Aids drug in Mainland China. *Asia Pacific Biotech, APBN*, Volume 5, Number 7.

Hong, H (2013). *Acupuncture: Theories and Evidence*. Singapore: World Scientific.

Huang Jianping (1995). *Methodology of Traditional Chinese Medicine*. Beijing: New World Press.

Johnston, I (Trans.) (2006). *Galen: On Diseases and Symptoms*. Cambridge: Cambridge University Press.

Julien, F (1995). *The Property of Things: Toward a History of Efficacy in China*. New York: Zone Books.

Kaptchuk, T (1998). Powerful placebo: The dark side of the randomised controlled trial. *Lancet*, 351: 1722–1725.

Kaptchuk, T (2000). *The Web that has no Weaver: Understanding Chinese Medicine*. New York: McGraw Hill.

Kendrick, M (17 July 2009). Anti-aging pill targets telomeres at the ends of chromosomes. *Scientific American*, 17 August 2009.

Kienle, G and Kiene, H (1997). The powerful placebo effect: Fact or fiction? *Journal of Clinical Epidemiology*, 50(12): 1311–1318.

Kleinman, A (1995). *Writing at the Margin: Discourse between Anthropology and Medicine.* Berkeley: University of California Press.

Krauss, L (2012). *A Universe From Nothing: Why There is Something Rather Than Nothing.* New York: Free Press.

Kuhn, T (1970). *The Structure of Scientific Revolutions,* Revised Edition. Chicago: Chicago University Press.

Kuhn, T (1974). Second thought on paradigms. Reprinted in *The Essential Tension,* Chicago, pp. 293–319 (1977).

Kuhn, T (1977). *The Essential Tension.* Chicago: University of Chicago Press.

Kuriyama, S (1999). *The Expressiveness of the Body.* New York: Zone Books.

Lai, SL (2001). *Clinical Trials of Traditional Chinese Materia Medica.* China: Guangdong People's Publishing House.

Lai, SL (2010). Meta-analysis of clinical trials. Unpublished paper presented at the *Annual Meeting of the Consortium for the Globalisation of Chinese Medicine (CGCM),* 24 August 2010.

Lakatos, I (1970). History of science and its rational reconstructions. *Proceedings of the Biennial Meeting of the Philosophy of Science Association,* pp. 91–136. Chicago: Chicago University Press.

Lei, S (1999). *When Chinese Medicine Encountered the State, 1910–1949.* Ph.D. Dissertation, University of Chicago.

Lei, S (2002). How did Chinese medicine become experiential? The political epistemology of Jingyan. *Positions,* 10(2): 335–338.

Leung, PC, Xue, CC and Cheng, CC (2003). *A Comprehensive Guide to Chinese Medicine.* Singapore: World Scientific.

Lewis, D (1973). Causation. Seventieth Annual Meeting of the American Philosophical Association Eastern Division (Oct. 11, 1973). *The Journal of Philosophy,* 70(17): 556–567.

Linde, K *et al.* (2005). Acupuncture for patients with migraine: A randomised controlled trial. *Journal of the American Medical Association,* 293: 2118–2125.

Linde, K *et al.* (2007). The impact of patient expectations on outcomes in four randomised controlled trials of acupuncture in patients with chronic pain. *Pain,* 128: 264–271.

Liu Lihong (2003). *Shikao Zhongyi* 思考中医 (*Thoughts on Chinese Medicine*), *Guangxi Daxue Chubanshe* (Guangxi University Press).

Lloyd, GER (Ed.) (1983). *Hippocratic Writings*. London: Penguin.

Lloyd, GER (1996). *Adversaries and Authorities*. Cambridge: Cambridge University Press.

Lloyd, GER (2003). *In the Grip of Disease*. Oxford: Oxford University Press.

Lloyd, GER (2006). *Principles and Practices in Ancient Greek and Chinese Science*. Hampshire: Ashgate.

Lloyd, GER and Sivin, N (2002). *The Way and the Word*. New Haven: Yale University Press.

Lo, V (2002). Introduction. In: G-D Lu and J Needham, *Celestial Lancets*. Reprinted by Routledge (1980).

Lo Yin (September 2004). What is *Qi*? Can we see *Qi*? *Acupuncture Today*, Volume 5, Issue 9.

Lu, AP, Liu, XW and Ding, XR (2009). Methodology of pharmacodynamic evaluation on Chinese herbal medicine based on syndrome differentiation. *Journal of Chinese Integrative Medicine*, 7(6): 501–504.

Lu, G-D and Needham, J (1980). *Celestial Lancets*. Reprinted by Routledge (2002).

Maxwell, G (1962). The Ontological Status of Theoretical Entities. Reprinted in Curd and Cover, *Philosophy of Science*, Norton (1998).

Melchart, D, Streng, A, Hoppe A, *et al.* (2005). Acupuncture in patients with tension-type headache: Randomised controlled trial. *British Medical Journal*, 331: 376–382.

Mestel, R (6 August 2001). Modern bloodletting and leeches. *Los Angeles Times*. Retrieved 17 December 2013. http://articles.latimes.com/2001/aug/06/health/he-31093.

Munson, R (1981). Why medicine cannot be a science. *The Journal of Medicine and Philosophy*, 6: 183–208.

Nagel, E (1961). *The Structure of Science: Problems in the Logic of Scientific Explanation*. New York: Harcourt, Brace & World.

National Cancer Institute (2013) *Helicobacter pylori* and cancer. Retrieved 17 December 2013, http://www.cancer.gov/cancertopics/factsheet/Risk/h-pylori-cancer.

National Cancer Institute (2011). *Helicobacter pylori* and cancer. Retrieved 17 December 2013. http://www.cancer.gov/cancertopics/factsheet/Risk/h-pylori-cancer.

Needham, J (1978). *The Shorter Science and Civilisation in China*, Volume II. Cambridge: Cambridge University Press.

Needham, J (2004). *Science and Civilisation in China*, Volume VI, Part VI. Cambridge: Cambridge University Press.

Needham, J and Lu, G-D (1975). Problems of translations and modernisation of ancient Chinese technical terms. *Annals of Science*, 32: 491–501.

Nickles, T (1998). Kuhn, historical philosophy of science, and case-based reasoning. *Configurations*, 6(1): 51–85.

Nickles, T (2003). Normal science: From logic to case-based and model-based. In: T Nickles (Ed.) *Thomas Kuhn*. Cambridge: Cambridge University Press.

Nisbett, R (2003). *The Geography of Thought*. New York: Free Press.

Nutton, V (2004). *Ancient Medicine*. London: Routledge.

Okasha, S (2002). *Philosophy of Science*. Oxford: OUP.

Ou Jiecheng 区结成 (2005). *Dang Zhongyi Yushang Xiyi* 当中医遇上西医 *(When Chinese Medicine Meets Western Medicine)*, Sanlian Shudian.

Oxford Concise Medical Dictionary (2007), 4th Edition. Oxford: Oxford University Press.

Peng Tian (2011). Convergence: Where west meets east. *Nature*, 480(7378): S84–S86.

Popper, K (2002). *The Logic of Scientific Discovery*. London: Routledge.

Porkert, M (1974). *Theoretical Foundations of Traditional Chinese Medicine*. Cambridge, MA: MIT Press.

Porter, R (1999). *The Greatest Benefit to Mankind: A Medical History of Humanity from Antiquity to the Present*. London: Fontana Press.

Psillos, S (2007). *Philosophy of Science A-Z*. Edinburgh: Edinburgh University Press.

Rawlins, MD (16 October 2008). On the evidence for decisions about the use of therapeutic interventions. Harvein Oration, Royal College of Physicians.

Reid, D (2001). *Traditional Chinese Medicine*. Periplus.

Ren Yingqiu 任应秋 (Ed.) (1986). *Zhongguo Gejia Xueshuo* (Schools of Thought in Chinese Medicine). *Shanghai Kexuejishu Chubanshe*.

Rosenberg, A (2005). *Philosophy of Science*. London: Routledge.

Rothman, KJ (2002). *Epidemiology*. Oxford: Oxford University Press.

Rothman, K and Greenland, S (2005). Causation and causal inference in epidemiology. *American Journal of Public Health*, 95: S144–S150.

Rudner, R (1953). The scientist *Qua* scientist makes value judgments. *Philosophy of Science*, 20: 1–6. Reprinted in Klemke, Hollinger and Rudge (1998) *Introductory Readings in the Philosophy of Science,* 3rd Edition. Promethus Books.

Sankey, H (2008). *Scientific Realism and the Rationality of Science.* Hampshire: Ashgate.

Sauer, U, Heinemann, M, and Zamboni, N (2007). GENETICS: Getting closer to the whole picture. *Science*, 316(5824): 550–551.

Schaffner, KF (1999). Philosophy of medicine. In: M Salmon *et al.* (Eds.) *Introduction to the Philosophy of Science.* Indianapolis: Hackett Publishing Co.

Scheid, V (2002). *Chinese Medicine in Contemporary China: Plurality and Synthesis.* North Carolina: Duke University Press.

Schwartz, V (1986). *The Chinese Enlightenment.* Berkeley: University of California Press.

Shahar, E (1988). Evidence-based medicine: A new paradigm or the Emperor's new clothes? *Journal of Evaluation in Clinical Practice*, 4(4): 227–282.

Shang, A, Huwiler, K *et al.* (2007). Placebo-controlled trials of Chinese herbal medicine and conventional medicine — comparative study. *International Journal of Epidemiology*, 36: 1086–1092.

Shea, JL (2006). Applying evidence-based medicine to traditional Chinese medicine: Debate and strategy. *Journal of Alternative and Complementary Medicine*, 12(3): 255–263.

Sinatra, S (2013). http://173.45.234.153/sinatra_staging/index.php/lower-lpa-with-5-nutrients.

Sinatra, ST (2012). Tumeric the super spice. Retrieved 17 December 2013. http://www.drsinatra.com/tumeric-super-spice.

Sinatra, ST and Roberts, JC (2007). *Reverse Heart Disease Now.* New Jersey: Wiley.

Singh, S and Ernst, E (2008). *Trick or Treatment? Alternative Medicine on Trial.* UK: Bantam.

Sivin, N (1987). *Traditional Medicine in Contemporary China.* Ann Arbor: University of Michigan Press.

Stanford Encyclopedia of Philosophy (2003). Teleological notions in biology. Retrieved 11 November 2012. http://plato.stanford.edu/entries/teleology-biology/.

Stebhens, WE (1992). Causality in medical science with particular reference to heart disease and arterosclerosis. *Perspectives in Biology and Medicine*, 36: 97–119.

Stevens, R (1983). *Law School: Legal Education in America from the 1850s to the 1980s.* Chapel Hill: University of North Carolina Press.

Taber's Cyclopedic Medical Dictionary (2001), 19th Edition. Philadelphia: F.A. Davis.

Tang Decai (2003). *Science of Chinese Materia Medica.* Shanghai University of Chinese Medicine Publishing House (in Chinese with English translation).

Tang, J-L (2006). Research priorities in traditional Chinese medicine. *British Medical Journal*, 333(7564): 391–394.

Tang, J-L, Zhan, S-Y and Ernst, E (1999). Review of randomised control trials of traditional Chinese medicine. *British Medical Journal*, 319: 160–161.

Taylor, K (2005). *Chinese Medicine in Early Communist China, 1945–1963.* New York: Routledge Curzon.

Tecusan, M (2004). *The Fragments of the Methodists.* Leiden: Brill.

Temkin, O and Temkin, CL (Eds.) (1967). *Ancient Medicine: Selected Papers of Ludwig Edelstein.* Baltimore: John Hopkins University Press.

Unschuld, P (1985). *Medicine in China: A History of Ideas.* Berkeley: University of California Press.

Unschuld, P (1989). *Approaches to Chinese Medical Literature.* Dordrecht: Kluwer Academic Publishers.

Unschuld, P (2003). *Huang Di Nei Jing Su Wen.* Berkeley: University of California Press.

Urbach, P (1985). Randomization and the design of experiments. *Philosophy of Science*, 52: 256–273.

van Frassen, B (1980). *The Scientific Image.* Oxford: Oxford University Press.

von Gyory, T (1905). *Semmelweis' Gesammelete Werke.* Jena: Gustav Fischer.

Wang Lufen (2002). *Diagnostics of Traditional Chinese Medicine.* Shanghai: Shanghai University of Chinese Medicine Press.

Wang, S *et al.* (2004). Angiogenesis and anti-angiogenesis activity of Chinese medicinal herbal extracts. *Life Science*, 74(20): 2467–2478.

Wang Xinhua 王新华 (Ed.) (2001). *Zhongyi Jichulun* 中医基础论 *(The Basic Theory of Traditional Chinese Medicine). Renmin Weisheng Chubanshe.*

Wang Yongyan 王永炎 (Ed.) (1998). *Zhongyi Neike Xue* 中医内科学 *(Chinese Internal Medicine)*. Shanghai: *Shangai Kexue Jishu Chubanshe*.

Wang Zhipu 王致谱 (2005). *Qun Jing Jian Zhi Lu* 群经见智路. *Fujian Kexue Jishu Chubanshe*.

Wang Zhongshang 王忠上 (2003). 从库恩的范式理论看中医学的发展 (The development of TCM from the point of view of Kuhn's theory of paradigms). 医学与社会 *(Medicine and Society)*. Beijing: Ministry of Education, Volume 16, Number 2.

Weil, A (1995). *Natural Health, Natural Medicine*. Houghton Mifflin.

WHO (World Health Organisation) (1985). *The Role of Traditional Chinese Medicine in Healthcare in Primary Health Care China*, Report of Seminar Proceedings 9–21 Oct, TRM/86.2, edited by O Akerele, G Stott and Weibo Lu.

WHO (2003). Acupuncture: Review and analysis of reports on controlled clinical trials. Retrieved 17 December 2013. http://apps.who.int/medicinedocs/en/d/Js4926e/5.html.

WHO Regional Office for the Western Pacific (2007). *WHO International Standard Terminologies on Traditional Medicine in the Western Pacific Region*.

Wiseman, N (2000). *Translation of Chinese Medical Terms: A Source-Oriented Approach*. Ph.D. Dissertation, University of Exeter.

Wiseman, N (2001). Translation of Chinese medical terms: Not just a matter of words. *Clinical Acupuncture and Oriental Medicine*, 2(1): 50–59.

Wiseman, N (2006). English translation of Chinese medicine: Concerning the use of Western medical terms to represent traditional Chinese medical concepts — Answer to Prof. Xie and his colleagues. *Chinese Journal of Integrative Medicine*, 12(3): 225.

Wiseman, N and Feng, Y (2002). *A Practical Dictionary of Chinese Medicine*, 2nd Edition. MA: Paradigm Publishers. Mandarin version published by *Renmin Weisheng Chubanshe*.

Witt, C, Brinkhaus, B, Jena, S *et al.* (2005). Acupuncture in patients with osteoarthritis of the knee: A randomised trial. *Lancet*, 366: 136–143.

Wittgenstein, L (1953). *Philosophical Investigations*. Oxford: Blackwell.

Worrall, J (2002). What evidence in evidence-based medicine? *Philosophy of Science*, 69: 316–330.

Worrall, J (2007). Why there's no cause to randomise. *British Medical Journal,* 58: 451–588.

Wu Changguo (Ed.) (2002). *Basic Theory of Traditional Chinese Medicine.* (In Chinese with English translation.) Shanghai University of Chinese Medicine Publishing House.

Wu Dunxu (Ed.) (1995). *Zhongyi Jichu Lilun.* Shanghai Science and Technology Press.

Wu Jing (2010). Placebo control and clinical trial of Chinese Medicine. *Journal of Integrative Chinese Medicine,* 8(10): 906–910.

Wu, N and Wu, A (Trans.) (1997). *Huangdi Neijing. The Yellow Emperor's Canon of Internal Medicine.* China: China Science and Technology Press.

Xie Zhufan (2003). *On Standard TCM Nomenclature.* Beijing: Foreign Languages Press.

Xie Zhufan (2004). *Translation of Common Terms in Traditional Chinese Medicine. Zhongguo Yiyao Chubanshe.*

Xie Zhufan *et al.* (2005). Comments on Nigel Wiseman's 'A Practical Dictionary of Chinese Medicine' — On Wiseman's literal translation. *Zhongguo Zhong Xi Yi Jie He Za Zhi,* 25(10): 937–940. (Article in Chinese with Abstract in English.)

Xie, Zhufan and White, P (2005). Comments on Nigel Wiseman's 'A Practical Dictionary of Chinese Medicine' — On the 'word-for-word' literal approach to translation. *Chinese Journal of Integrative Medicine,* 11(4): 305–308.

Xin, B (2003). More theories about acupuncture. In: PC Leung, CC Xie and CC Cheng (Eds.) *A Comprehensive Guide to Chinese Medicine.* Singapore: World Scientific.

Yellow Emperor's Canon of Medicine (2005). Translated by Li Zhaoguo. Xi'an: World Publishing Corporation.

Yu Rencun and Hong Hai (2012). *Cancer Management with Chinese Medicine.* Singapore: World Scientific.

Yu Yan 余岩 (1933). '*Ling Su Shang Dui* 灵素商兑'. In: *Yixue Geming Lun* 医学革命论初集 *(Treatise on Revolution in Medical Thought).* Shanghai: The Commercial Press. The exact date of Yu Yan's paper is not available, although it clearly was printed and circulated before 1922 and published only later.

Yun Tieqiao 恽铁樵 (1922). "*Qun Jing Jian Zhi Lu*" 《群经见智录》in 《论医集.对于改进中医之意见》.

Zhang Gongyao 王功耀 (2006). Farewell to traditional Chinese medicine. *Medicine and Philosophy*, 27(4): 14–17.

Zhang Jie (2005). 利用方证相应学说探寻中医证的物质基础 (Examining the concept of syndrome by correspondence between syndrome and prescription). *Journal of the China Academy of Chinese Medical Sciences*, 12(11): 3–5.

Zhang Jun 张军 (1 September 2005). 论任应秋阴阳五行观对现代中医发展的影响 (On Ren Yingqiu's views on yin-yang and five phases on the development of modern TCM). 德明中医.

Zhang Qicheng (1996). *Lun Zhongyi Siwei Ji Qi Zouxiang* 论中医思维及其走向. 中国中医基础杂志 (*Journal of Chinese Medical Foundations*), 2(4): 10–12.

Zhang Qicheng (1999). *Moxing Yu Yuanxing: Zhong Xi Yi De Benzhi Qubie* 模型与原型：中西医的本质区别. 西学与哲学 (*Medicine and Philosophy*), 12(8): 213–227.

Zheng Xian (1985). Observation of 42 cases of entero-susceptible syndrome treated by traditional Chinese medicine differentiation of symptoms and signs. *Journal of Traditional Chinese Medicine*, 26(2): 36–37.

Zhongguo dabaikequanshu: Zhongyi 中国大百科全书: 中医 (*The Chinese Encyclopedia: Chinese Medicine volume*) (2001). Entry on "Qi", pp. 238–239. Beijing: *Zhongguo dabaikequanshu chubanshe.*

Zhou Zhong Ying (2007). *Zhongyi Neike Xue* 中医内科学. Beijing: *Zhongguo zhongyiyao chuban she.*

Zhu Qing Shi (Ed.) (2005). *Zheyan Kan Zhongyi* 哲眼看中医 (Chinese medicine viewed from the philosopher's eye). 北京科学技术出版社. Beijing Science and Technology Press.

Index

Printed in the United States
By Bookmasters